Practice Nurse Handbook

Practice Nurse Handbook

Fourth edition

Gillian Hampson
RGN, RCNT, DN, PN/dip HE in community health care
Practice Nurse, Chartfield Surgery, Putney

Blackwell
Science

© 2002 by Blackwell Science Ltd,
a Blackwell Publishing Company
Editorial Offices:
Osney Mead, Oxford OX2 0EL, UK
 Tel: +44 (0)1865 206206
Blackwell Science, Inc., 350 Main Street,
Malden, MA 02148-5018, USA
 Tel: +1 781 388 8250
Iowa State Press, a Blackwell Publishing
Company, 2121 State Avenue, Ames, Iowa
50014-8300, USA
 Tel: +1 515 292 0140
Blackwell Publishing Asia Pty Ltd,
550 Swanston Street, Carlton South, Melbourne,
Victoria 3053, Australia
 Tel: +61 (0)3 9347 0300
Blackwell Wissenschafts Verlag,
Kurfürstendamm 57, 10707 Berlin, Germany
 Tel: +49 (0)30 32 79 060

First edition published 1984
Second edition published 1989
Reprinted 1989
Third edition published 1994,
Fourth edition published 2002

Library of Congress
Cataloging-in-Publication Data
is available

ISBN 0-632-06392-0

A catalogue record for this title is available from
the British Library

Set in 10/12.5 Palatino
by DP Photosetting, Aylesbury, Bucks
Printed and bound in Great Britain by
MPG Books Ltd, Bodmin, Cornwall

For further information on
Blackwell Science, visit our website:
www.blackwell-science.com

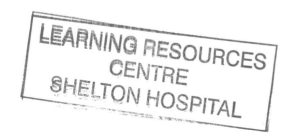

Contents

Contributors

CHAPTER 3
Susan Wilson (Computers)
IM & T Manager, Richmond PCG

CHAPTER 4
Chrissy Tinson (Control of infection)
Practice Nurse Adviser, Infection Control

CHAPTER 5
Hilary Harkin (Ear care)
Primary Ear Care Trainer
Primary Ear Care Training Centre, Rotherham

CHAPTER 6
Hilary Magill (Diagnostic tests and investigations)
Senior Practitioner, Practice Nursing
Chrissy Tinson
Practice Nurse Adviser, Infection Control

CHAPTER 9
Jenny MacLeod (Healthy eating)
Dietitian, Queen Mary's Hospital, Roehampton and Kingston Hospital

CHAPTER 10
Veronique Gibbons
Immunisation Advice Nurse, PHLS

CHAPTER 11
Mary Lowe (Travel health)
Clinical Governance Facilitator

CHAPTER 15
Nesta Jones (Men's health)
Specialist Practitioner, General Practice Nursing,
Chartfield Surgery, Putney

CHAPTER 16
Ingrid Clarke (Diabetes)
Diabetes Liaison Nurse, Richmond PCG
Margaret Lyons (Heart disease)
Cardiac Nurse Specialist, Richmond PCG

Preface to the Fourth Edition

So many changes have happened in practice nursing and within the National Health Service since writing the last edition in 1994, that it was difficult to decide how to proceed. The nursing journals frequently contain articles about the pioneering work of individual practice nurses, which make other experiences seem humble by comparison. In deciding what information to include, I tried to think of those things I most needed to know when new to practice nursing. I adopted the same objectives as last time. Namely: to give as many practical hints and pointers as possible, to draw attention to the legal pitfalls, and to indicate ways that practice nurses can develop their role. The emphasis throughout is on the need for on-going education.

The Internet has been invaluable in verifying facts and seeking new information. I have included many of the web sites which were particularly useful. The sheer scale of the information available and the volume of Government documents online, has meant that this book has assumed a rather Anglo-centric nature. I hope that readers in other parts of the United Kingdom will forgive this.

Gillian Hampson

Acknowledgement

Nesta Jones also generously gave her time to provide constructive criticism about other chapters and helped with finding reference material, even while she was studying successfully for her BSc degree in practice nursing. Her assistance was greatly appreciated.

Chapter 1
Teamwork in General Practice

This chapter outlines the background to the work of practice nurses so that their role can considered within the context of the whole primary health care team.

The National Health Service (NHS)

In 1948 the National Health Service was established on the basis that everybody should have free access to medical care irrespective of their financial state. It seems naive now, to realise that at that time it was assumed that the demand for care would decrease once the unresolved 'pool' of illness in the population had been treated. In the light of experience it has become clear that the amount of treatable illness is small, compared with either chronic conditions which cannot be cured, or the problems created by environmental and personal stress; the underlying reasons for many consultations in general practice.

Developments in general practice

Prior to 1948 most general practitioners worked independently; usually from their own homes. Patients who were unable to afford private medical care belonged to a doctor's panel. The cost was supported by various insurance schemes, and hospital beds were endowed especially for 'the poor'. The hospitals were nationalised in 1948, but general practitioners, dentists, retail pharmacists and opticians stayed as independent businesses with contracts to supply specific services to NHS patients. Executive Councils were set up to administer these arrangements. District nurses and health visitors were employed by the local authorities.

The early days of the NHS were a catalogue of disasters, with neither doctors nor patients really knowing what to expect of the new system. Patients had been led to believe that everything was free; so extra demands were made upon doctors, who were themselves unprepared for the organisational and practical difficulties created by the new system. Between 1948 and 1956 expenditure in the NHS had risen by 70%[1].

The Family Doctors' Charter

The British Medical Association, through its General Medical Services Committee, has always been responsible for the political aspects of general practice. This includes terms of service and remuneration. The College of General Practitioners, established in 1953 (to become the Royal College in 1966), was mainly concerned with educational issues. The effects of these two bodies on government policies brought about in 1966 the so-called *GPs' Charter*, in response to the threat of resignation by disillusioned doctors[2]. The Charter radically altered the way in which GPs were paid and gave them incentives for having better premises and reimbursement for ancillary staff salaries. Nurses were included among these ancillary staff, which may account for some of the attitudes subsequently displayed towards nurses employed in general practice.

NHS reorganisation

The structure of the NHS was reorganised in 1974, when management first assumed a specialist function. Executive councils became family practitioner committees (FPCs) and community nurse employment was transferred from local authorities to the health service. Area health authorities were abolished in 1982 and their powers devolved to district health authorities. However, 1990 saw a more radical change to the NHS. The introduction of the internal market created a separation between the purchasers and the providers of services. Hospitals were invited to become self-governing trusts and GPs in group practices were encouraged to become fund-holders to purchase secondary services on behalf of their patients. FPCs were changed to family health service authorities (FHSAs) with greater managerial responsibilities in relation to general practice[3]. FHSAs later merged with health authorities and some of their functions were devolved to primary care agencies (PCAs).

A change of government in 1997 led to the development of *The New NHS*[4]. Fund-holding was abolished and instead of being in competition, all the practices in a locality became part of primary care groups. These were subcommittees of health authorities, with a devolved budget to purchase services on behalf of the local community and a remit to monitor and improve the quality of services (clinical governance) and promote improvements in health (health improvement programmes). The pace of change became unremitting, with a stream of targets to reduce waiting lists and national service frameworks (NSFs) specifying standards for services for the common diseases. The National Institute for Clinical Excellence was established to make recommendations on the use of new drugs and treatments in order to end the 'postcode lottery', whereby patients in one health authority area could be denied treatments available elsewhere. The Commission for Health Improvement was established to inspect health authorities and trusts (including general practices) and to monitor performance. The National Clinical Assessment Authority was set up to provide a rapid investigation into the performance of certain doctors, in the wake of several medical scandals[5-7].

The NHS plan

In the year 2000 the Government published an ambitious plan for investment and reform of the NHS to take place over ten years[8]. The plan outlined the intention to provide extra beds, hospitals and staff, as well as modernisation of general practice, new doctors' contracts and a greater role for nurses. The role of patients in the modernisation process was also stressed.

Primary care trusts (PCTs)

Primary care trusts quickly replaced PCGs; becoming autonomous providers of general practice and community nursing services and commissioners of secondary care. As many of the functions of the health authorities have been devolved to PCTs, health authorities have started to merge into larger strategic bodies akin to the old regional health authorities. Proposals are also contained in the NHS plan for PCTs to merge with social service departments to form care trusts, with budgets to provide integrated health and social services.

Health Service structures

Although politics can seem remote from direct patient care, it is essential to keep abreast of developments in the organisation of the NHS. Nurses have a key role to play in the changing NHS and in developing innovative services and ways of promoting health for the public.

The structures for Scotland, Wales and Northern Ireland were always slightly different but there are likely to be more significant changes now that parliamentary devolution has taken place. The NHS Policy Board decides the overall strategy for the NHS. The various directorates and branches of the NHS Executive (NHSE) are responsible for the operation of the service in terms of effectiveness and value for money.

The 'New' GP Contract

In 1990 the Government imposed a new contract on GPs; requiring them to provide a range of screening and health promotion services. Many practice nurses were employed at that time to undertake the extra work[9]. Apart from the medical services already offered to patients, the new contract required GPs to be responsible for:

- Child health surveillance – developmental checks up to the age of five for which a single fee may be claimed
- Registration health checks – for all patients aged 5–75 (a fee can be claimed)

- Annual health checks for patients aged over 75 years
- Health promotion clinics (clinic fees were replaced in 1993 by target payments for specific health promotion activities)
- Minor surgery – by doctors accepted onto the minor surgery list (fees can be claimed for 15 minor operations per GP each quarter).

Health targets

In that same year, the Government introduced targets for reducing disease and disability through its *Health of the Nation* strategy for England. This was replaced in 1997 by the Labour Government's strategy document *Saving Lives: The Nation's Health*[10]. Similar strategies were produced in the other countries of Great Britain.

Care in the community

Other changes accelerated within the community from April 1993 as a result of the NHS and Community Care Act (1990). Social service departments assumed new responsibilities for assessing the needs and providing tailor-made services for vulnerable people. Hospitals had to ensure that the appropriate services were in place before such patients could be discharged home. More resources were needed to provide effective community care and plans were made to modernise mental health services[11]. *The National Service Framework for Mental Health*, published in 1999, was intended to address some of the failings of care in the community (see Chapter 15).

General practice as a business

Unlike hospital doctors, who are salaried, GPs have always been independent contractors, with the same contract with the NHS for providing general medical services (GMS). This has a very complicated system of remuneration and *The Statement of Fees and Allowances* (known as the Red Book) gives details of all the payments which GPs may receive from the NHS. Payments include:

- Basic practice allowance – towards the costs incurred in providing medical services to NHS patients.
- Capitation fees – for each patient registered. Higher rates are paid for patients aged over 65 and over 75 years of age, to reflect the increased healthcare needs of older people. Higher rates are also paid for the extra work generated in areas of social deprivation (calculated using the Jarman Index of Deprivation[12]).
- Item of service fees – can be claimed for additional services, e.g. family planning, registration health checks, some immunisation. (Payments for cervical screening and childhood immunisation may sometimes only be

made when overall targets are reached.) Maternity care, night visits and emergency treatment can attract fees.
- Other payments
  - Budgets include partial reimbursement for ancillary staff salaries and training costs.
  - Other diverse activities, such as teaching medical students or dispensing, may earn payments.
  - The postgraduate education allowance (PGEA) is paid to doctors who provide the required evidence of professional updating. The system for managing PGEA is being updated.

Apart from payments by the NHS, GPs are entitled to charge for activities not covered by their contract, such as writing reports, private medical certificates and examinations, or for treating non-NHS patients privately. PCTs may now give additional incentive payments for effective prescribing and meeting clinical governance and HlmP targets, or provide money for practice development schemes.

Personal medical services (PMS)

The Primary Care Act of 1997 permitted a departure from the national GMS contract[13]. PMS pilot practices (the first wave started in 1998), demonstrated new ways of providing general practice services, through local contracts with health authorities (later with primary care trusts). Some pilots have been led by nurses, who employ salaried GPs to provide medical services to their practice populations. The majority of nurse-led pilots have tended to provide services for specific population groups, such as the homeless, refugees and asylum seekers; or people in under-doctored areas[14].

Education

Postgraduate training for general practice was introduced on a more formal basis in 1973, followed by the Vocational Training Act in 1981. It is now impossible to become a principal in general practice without three years specific postgraduate education, which includes one year as a registrar in an approved training practice. However, many changes are in the offing for all professional education. Multi-professional education, whereby members of different professions learn together and are able to switch more easily between career pathways has been strongly advocated by the Department of Health[15]. Workforce development confederations have taken the place of the local medical workforce advisory groups and the education consortia in order to bring all the branches of health-related professional education under one umbrella. The inclusion of patients in education for the professions is a welcome part of the move to involve the public more closely in the running of the NHS.

Revalidation

The General Medical Council has instituted a process of appraisals for GPs, who will be required to develop personal learning plans and to demonstrate their fitness to practice. Revalidation at regular intervals may also be required[16]. Practice development plans are a way of ensuring all practice staff reach their full potential and that lifelong learning underpins the work of everybody. Nurses are already accustomed to keeping professional profiles and to reregistering every three years. The terminology used for development varies from area to area, so the use of abbreviations can be misleading. In some areas personal development plans may be confused with practice development plans if both are called PDPs.

Beacon practices

Practices which have demonstrated particular expertise or have developed innovative ways of working can be registered as beacon practices, which members of other practices can visit to learn about their successes and problems[17]. A booklet is available listing the beacon sites and the reason beacon status was awarded.

Practice population profiles

The changes within the NHS necessitate the identification of the particular health and social needs of local populations in order to provide appropriate services. Such profiles should cover: age/sex ratios, ethnic groups, family structures, numbers on the child protection register, social class, poverty levels, employment, housing, vulnerable groups, morbidity and mortality, environmental hazards and amenities. Since April 2000 practices have also been required to identify all informal carers registered with them, whether or not the person for whom they care is registered at the same practice[18]. Practices have a duty to ensure that carers are offered the support and help to which they are entitled.

Teamwork

The explosion of work within general practice highlights the need for good teamwork, but just being together in one place will not create a team. All teams share certain characteristics, whatever their functions:

- A shared purpose or goal
- A sense of team identity
- An understanding of the role and valuing of the contribution of individual team members.

Teamwork needs some committed hard work to succeed. It can be hindered by ineffective leadership, divided loyalties when members belong to more than one team, or sabotage by disaffected members.

The historical background to the different professions means that modern-day, independent-minded nurses, and GPs accustomed to assume authority, may have very different perceptions of the same situation. The importance of team-building has been recognised for many years in the commercial world and many of their methods are being adopted in the health service.

Primary healthcare

Primary healthcare refers to health promotion and care within general practice and the community, as compared with secondary care provided by hospitals and specialist services. The Government is investing extra money to promote primary care services[19]. Primary healthcare teams have been around since the 1960s in one guise or another, but in reality there are often two types of team involved with general practice.

The practice team

A practice team tends to incorporate all those people based within the practice; most of whom are either partners, or directly employed by the GP. Apart from the doctors, practice teams include:

The practice nurse(s) (see Chapter 2)   The title, *practice nurse*, has always been generally understood to apply to a qualified nurse employed directly by a GP or GP partnership. A practice may also include a nurse practitioner in the team, although the qualification and title is not yet protected by the UKCC and the work undertaken is subject to wide variations[20].

The practice manager   A practice manager has responsibility for organising the systems which allow the practice to run smoothly and to provide a high quality service to the patients, as well as for financial and personnel management, staff development and liaison with all the staff and the PCT. The original practice managers were often senior receptionists, for whom this was a logical pro-motion. However, a new breed of practice manager has emerged, with the specific management training needed; often a university degree in business management.

The receptionists   The receptionists are the first point of contact with the public. They must be able to stay calm in the face of conflicting demands from patients, other staff and the telephone. Receptionists frequently act as gatekeepers to the doctors and nurses by prioritising appointments or controlling the number of telephone calls put through. A very fine line exists between efficient organi-sation and denial of a patient's right to consult a doctor or nurse.

Apart from running the appointment system and taking telephone messages, there is plenty of administrative work. Most practices are computerised and registration data has to be processed. Some receptionists organise repeat prescriptions and help to process fee claims. Filing clerks prepare the records for surgery sessions and file letters, reports and the patients' records after use. Data entry clerks type data into the computers. Training for receptionists often takes place in-house but recognised courses are also available. Practice receptionist training, organised by some PCTs and colleges of further education, leads to a qualification from the Association of Medical Secretaries and Practice Managers, Administrators and Receptionists (AMSPAR).

The medical secretary   A medical secretary needs office skills and a knowledge of the terminology used in medical correspondence. In smaller practices secretarial duties may be combined with reception or administrative work, but large practices usually employ a qualified medical secretary to deal specifically with referral letters, reports, office administration and the practice correspondence.

Paramedical staff   Larger practices may employ or facilitate access to other professional staff – dietitians, physiotherapists, counsellors and chiropodists, to increase the range of services available for patients. Pharmacists are joining many practices to help with more effective prescribing. Alternative therapists such as acupuncturists, aromatherapists and masseurs are also being welcomed into some teams.

Phlebotomists   Larger practices often employ a phlebotomist to take routine blood tests. In some areas, a member of the clerical staff has been trained in phlebotomy in order to free up valuable nursing time.

The primary healthcare team (PHCT)

Group attachment allows for better communication between the professional groups than when nurses work in geographical patches. District nurses, health visitors, community midwives and community mental health nurses also relate to teams in their own specialities, which may have different aims and priorities from those of the practice. Practice nurses are unique among NHS nurses in being employed by a GP and not by a community or hospital trust. It is possible that in the future, practice nurses, district nurses and health visitors will all be employed by the same local primary care trust.

Integrated nursing teams   The idea that community nurse attachment to GP practices would lead to integrated primary care teams has only rarely been realised fully. There have been a number of successful teams created in recent years consisting of district nurses, health visitors and practice nurses; some practices have been awarded beacon status because of their integrated nursing. The success of such teams often seems to rely on the degree of self-direction and budget-control permitted, as well as on the personalities of the team members themselves. The need to avoid duplication or gaps in the service is likely to lead to closer integration in the future and a radical rethink of the way nursing services are delivered.

Specialist community nurses

Since 1994 eight branches of community nursing have been accorded equal recognition by the UKCC, with recordable qualifications in specialist practice. Modules in common core subjects as well as discipline-specific modules in each of the specialties lead to a BSc or honours degree in one of the eight specialist fields:

- General practice nursing
- Community mental health nursing
- Community learning disabilities nursing
- Community children's nursing
- Public health nursing/health visiting
- School nursing
- Community nursing in the home/district nursing
- Occupational health nursing.

District nurses   A district nurse is responsible for providing skilled nursing services in the community by:

- Assessing the care needs of patients and their families
- Formulating individualised care plans and revising them as necessary
- Implementing the care or delegating to other members of the district nursing team
- Monitoring the patients' progress and reassessing care needs
- Supervising the care given by other members of the district nursing team.

Liaison with other PHCT members, social services and voluntary agencies is often as important as direct care-giving. The role also includes providing support to carers and teaching patients, other nurses and medical students. District nursing teams work in a similar way to hospital ward teams, with mixed skills and grades. Most district nursing care takes place within the patients' homes, although some district nurses also run clinics within health centres or general practices, e.g. leg ulcer clinics.

Health visitors   The role of health visitors is in a state of change. Health visiting evolved in the Victorian era to promote the welfare of mothers and children. Many health visitors still devote a high proportion of their time to work with the under-fives and to child protection work. However, the role can encompass health promotion with people of all ages and the importance of the public health role has also been reasserted in recent years.[21] Health visitors are developing many innovative ways of improving the health and welfare of their clients; ranging from working with young offenders to promoting the health and well-being of Asian men[22-3]. As with the district nurses, teaching and liaison with other agencies are also important aspects of the role of health visitors.

Community midwives   Midwives have statutory responsibilities for the care of women during pregnancy, confinement and the puerperium.[24] Community midwives organise antenatal and post-natal care and run ante-natal and parentcraft classes. A community midwife must attend a home confinement, and be responsible for a domino scheme or delivery within a GP hospital maternity unit. The midwife will care for a mother and baby up to the twenty eighth day after delivery and notify the health visitor when they are discharged. The *Midwifery Action Plan* proposes a broader role for midwives in women's health and public health and envisages extending the midwife's role in post-natal care.[25]

Other nurses may be considered as peripheral members of the PHCT. Each has a specific contribution to make, but the links with general practice are often more tenuous.

Community mental health nurses (CMHNs) – previously called community psychiatric nurses (CPNs) – are registered mental health nurses, who have undertaken post-registration studies in their field of expertise. The service developed out of hospital-based psychiatric nursing, and most CMHNs continue to be based in hospitals within community mental health teams. CMHNs carry out mental health assessments, support patients and their families within the community, and offer a range of therapeutic strategies (see Chapter 15, Mental Health).

School nurses have a major role in health promotion for school children, as well as in dealing with their health problems at school. School nurses carry out wide-scale immunisation programmes for school-age children and play a key role in helping to reduce the number of teenage pregnancies through sex education and the provision of practical advice. Practice nurses may have most contact with school nurses through the care of children with asthma or other chronic conditions.

Community children's nurses care for children with acute and chronic illnesses in their homes and provide valuable support for families. The children's nurses roles range from teaching wet-wrapping for eczema, to managing a terminal illness at home. Their degree of contact with the practice nurse can depend on the local arrangements.

Community learning disability nurses help people with learning disabilities to maximise their potential for independent living within the community. They help clients and carers to deal with physical, mental and social problems, including challenging behaviour, and liaise with a range of support services.

Hospital and community-based specialist nurses are a valuable resource for advice and teaching on their individual subjects – e.g. diabetes, continence, stoma care, HIV/AIDS, and infection control. Macmillan nurses provide a valuable service and may also be considered to be members of the extended healthcare team.

Social services

Referrals can be made on behalf of patients who require home care, meals on wheels, occupational therapy or other social service support. However, relatively few practices have a social worker attached and referrals for social services are usually made by telephone or letter. Social workers are expected to make a full needs assessment of the patients referred to them, although the National Service Framework for Older People requires health and social services to work together to ensure that single assessments of needs are carried out.[26]

Health visitors and GPs are sometimes involved with social workers on child protection issues. Also, an approved social worker is needed when a patient is compulsorily detained under the Mental Health Act (see Chapter 15).

Voluntary services

A huge number of voluntary services, self-help groups and charities exist. They provide financial and practical assistance, as well as information, advice and research funding. Some are organised locally to help people in need in that community, while others are organised nationally to help sufferers of a specific illness or disability. Patients and their carers can benefit from the knowledge of a practice nurse who can tell them who to approach for help. A database of contact addresses and web sites can be very useful, but it needs to be regularly updated. *E-MIMS*, available on CD-ROM and updated monthly, has details of most support groups as well as the drug information.

Some practices have a League of Friends, who organise voluntary transport, collect prescriptions, visit elderly or bereaved patients and even raise funds to buy special equipment for the practice. This type of voluntary work can provide significant help in both urban and rural communities.

Involvement of the public is one of the key elements of the plan for modernising the NHS. PCT boards have several lay non-executive members, and practices are expected to seek the opinions of patients about the quality of their services.

Suggestions for reflection on practice

- How much do you know about the way your local NHS is run? Who are the nurse leaders?
- How integrated is your PHC nursing team? What changes could be made to improve the service to patients?
- What does the health profile of your practice population reveal? Which groups of people need the most help?
- How easy is it to find out about the statutory and voluntary services available locally?
- How much involvement do patients have in the organisation of your practice? What changes could be made?

Further reading

Atkin, K., Lunt, N. and Thompson, C. (1999) *Evaluating Community Nursing*. Bailliere Tindall, London.

Craig, P. and Lindsay, G.M. (2000) *Nursing for Public Health. Population-based Care*. Churchill Livingstone, Edinburgh.

Department of Health (2001) *Health Improvement and Modernisation Plans – Guidance and Legislation. www.doh.gov.uk/himp/himpguidelegis*

Kesby, S. (2000) From reforms to modernisation. *Nursing Standard*, **15**(4), 40–6.

NHS Confederation (2000) *A Vision for Primary Care. Applying the modernisation approach*. NHS Confederation, Birmingham.

Pietroni, R. (2001) *The Toolbox for Portfolio Development*. Radcliffe Medical Press, Oxon.

Royal College of Nursing (2001) *Primary Care Trusts in England: the knowledge and skills nurses need to make them work*. Royal College of Nursing, London.

References

1. Allsop, J. (1984) *Health Policy and the National Health Service*. Longman, Harlow.
2. Ministry of Health (Gillie, A., Chairman) (1963) *The Field of Work of the Family Doctor*. HMSO, London.
3. Parliament (1990) *The National Health Service and Community Care Act 1990*. HMSO, London.
4. Department of Health (1997) *The New NHS: modern, dependable*. HMSO, London.
5. Department of Health (2001) *Harold Shipman's Clinical Practice 1974–97: a clinical audit commissioned by the Chief Medical Officer*. Department of Health, London.
6. Command Paper: Om5207 (2001) *Learning from Bristol: the report of the public enquiry into children's heart surgery at Bristol Royal Infirmary 1984–95*. Department of Health, London.

7. Department of Health (2000) *Consent to Organ and Tissue Retention at Post-mortem Examination and the Disposal of Human Tissue Materials.* HMSO, London.
8. Department of Health (2000) *The NHS Plan. A plan of investment. A plan for reform.* Department of Health, London.
9. Atkin, A., Lunt, K., Parker, G. & Hurst, M. (1993) *Nurses Count: a national census of practice nurses.* Social Policy Research Unit, University of York.
10. Department of Health (1999) *Saving Lives: Our Healthier Nation.* Department of Health, London.
11. Department of Health (1998) *Modernising Mental Health: Safe, Sound and Supportive.* Department of Health, London.
12. Jarman, B. (1983) Identification of underprivileged areas. *British Medical Journal*, **268**: 1705–09.
13. Parliament (1997) *National Health Service (Primary Care) Act 1997.* HMSO, London.
14. Lewis, R. (2001) *Nurse-led Primary Care. Learning from PMS pilots.* King's Fund Publishing, London.
15. Department of Health (2000) *A Health Service of All the Talents: developing the NHS workforce.* Department of Health, London.
16. General Medical Council (2000) *Proposals for Revalidation.* General Medical Council, London.
17. HSC 1999/034 (1999) *Beacon Primary Care Services.* Department of Health, London.
18. Department of Health (1999) *Caring about Carers: a national strategy for carers.* Department of Health, London.
19. Department of Health (2001) *Primary Care. Investing in Primary Care, www.doh.gov.uk/pricare/investment.* (accessed 4/8/01)
20. Lewis, R. (2001) *Nurse-led Primary Care. Learning from PMS pilots.* King's Fund Publishing, London.
21. Standing Nursing and Midwifery Advisory Committee (1995) *Making it Happen.* Department of Health, London.
22. Wildbore, A. (2001) Health and crime. *Community Practitioner*, **74** (8), 297.
23. Daniel, K. (2001) Damja breaks new ground. *Community Practitioner*, **74** (7), 255–6.
24. United Kingdom Central Council (1998) *Midwives Rules and Code of Practice.* United Kingdom Central Council, London.
25. Department of Health (2001) *'Making a Difference – the nursing, midwifery and health visiting contribution'. The Midwifery Action Plan.* Department of Health, London.
26. Department of Health (2001) *National Service Framework for Older People.* Department of Health, London.
27. Department of Health (1997) *The New NHS: modern, dependable.* Department of Health, London.

Useful addresses and web sites

Beacon practices
Web site *www.nhs.beacons.org.uk*

Department of Health
Richmond House, 79 Whitehall, London SW1A 2NS
Web site: *www.doh.gov.uk*

NHS Executive
Quarry House, Quarry Hill, Leeds LS2 7UE
Telephone: 0113 254 5610
Web site *www.doh.gov.uk/nhsexec/* (for details of regional offices)

NHS Modernisation Agency
Web site *www.modernnhs.nhs.uk*

Chapter 2
General Practice Nursing

One of the attractions of practice nursing is the flexibility it allows. Progressive nurses have blossomed in the atmosphere of general practice, and some have become celebrities through their innovations in health promotion and chronic disease management. But herein lies a dilemma, because that same flexibility can also lead to a diversity of standards.

Clinical governance is intended to iron out variations in quality. It is the modern term for the framework covering all the activities which contribute to a high quality service. This includes: education, risk assessment, evidence-based practice and audit, as well as patient feedback and the analysis of critical incidents and mistakes. The Royal College of Nursing has produced a useful guide for nurses on clinical governance[1].

Historical background

Practice nursing evolved over time; partly from the work of GPs' wives who were nurses and partly from district nurse attachment to general practice. The Health Services and Public Health Act (1968) gave the seal of approval for district nurses to extend their work to seeing patients in health centres and GP premises.

More practice nurses began to be employed by doctors in the early 1970s when it became apparent that the district nurses were unable to spend as long in the surgery, doing tasks like dressings and injections, as the doctors were asking them to do. One solution to this was for doctors to employ nurses directly. After 1966, when salaries could be partially reimbursed, practice nurses were classified with secretaries and receptionists as ancillary staff on the Family Practitioner Committee returns. Even as late as 1992, when asked by the Social Policy Research Unit to furnish the names of practice nurses for the National Census, some family health service authorities could not identify all the nurses in post[2].

Neighbourhood nursing

The Cumberlege Report in 1986 caused outrage to many practice nurses when it was suggested that all community nurses should be employed in neighbourhood nursing teams[3]. This concept of integrated nursing was not received with great joy by practice nurses. The proposal led to a new sense of group identity as practice nurses came together to fight for the right to continue being employed within general practice. The apparently illogical preference by members of one profession to be employed by members of another, owed much to the negative feelings felt by many practice nurses towards inflexible management in the NHS at that time.

Nurse education

The 1990 GP Contract led to a doubling, seemingly overnight, of the number of practice nurses employed[4]. This phenomenon caused a stir in nursing circles and concern at the lack of professional control over such a large group of nurses[5]. Practice nurse education finally began to receive serious attention. Practice nurses were suddenly overwhelmed by educational opportunities from a variety of sources but there was no simple way of assessing the quality of the education, and the amount of study leave granted to practice nurses varied from one practice to another. Nurse advisers/facilitators were appointed by many FHSAs to coordinate practice nurse education.

Project 2000 changed the traditional nurse training into a higher education system comparable with that of other disciplines[6]. Initially it was expected that this would equip nurses to work in any setting but it became obvious that more education would be needed for work in the community. The United Kingdom Central Council (UKCC) decision on community education finally gave qualified practice nurses and other community nurses equality with district nurses and health visitors as specialist practitioners (see Chapter 1, Teamwork in General Practice).

Practice nurses

The diversity of the work undertaken by practice nurses makes a precise description of the role very difficult. A recent study in Sheffield found both a seasonal variation and a wide range in the nursing activities and the time spent on them by individual nurses[7].

Treatment room nurses to healthcare assistants

Treatment room nurses were originally employed by the NHS for nursing work within health centres. They were not employed directly by the general practitioners. Few treatment room nurse posts exist nowadays but healthcare assistants (HCAs) are being employed in larger practices; they undertake some of the basic administrative, organisational and treatment room work previously undertaken by practice nurses. HCAs are able to study for national vocational qualifications (NVQs) to equip them for the role; by a distance learning programme if preferred. This example of skill mix allows a practice to make the best use of the time and expertise of its nurses.

Practice nurses

Practice nurses usually have a wide remit, although some practice nursing still contains an element of treatment room work. Practice nursing can be considered under several headings.

Management   This includes:

- Organising the nurses' rooms and work, including call/recall for health promotion
- Ensuring clinical stocks and supplies are maintained
- Collaboration on organisational and professional issues, including policies, protocols, quality standards and educational needs.

Clinical   This includes:

- Assessing patients' care needs
- Planning, providing, and evaluating the care given (this includes technical and nursing procedures as well as screening, and chronic disease management).

Communication   This includes:

- Giving information, support and advice to patients and carers; counselling and health promotion
- Liaison with other members of the practice team, the primary health care team, social services and other agencies
- Teaching patients, other nurses and students.

Audit and research   This includes:

- Compiling statistics and reports on nursing activities
- Identifying ways to improve nursing practice.

Because the work of practice nurses is so varied and challenging, it increases the need for up-to-date knowledge. Many practices have a practice library which should include a nursing section. There are many journals relevant to practice nursing (see Appendix 2). Information is available on the core competencies and personal development in *A Toolkit for Practice Nurses*[8].

Nurse practitioners

Nurse practitioners are experienced nurses who may have undertaken further specialised education at degree level to be able to work autonomously in a variety of settings. Examination skills and the management of injury or diseases, traditionally the prerogative of doctors, are among the subjects taught on nurse practitioner courses. However, because the title is not recordable with the UKCC, there is nothing to stop a nurse from calling him/herself a nurse practitioner by virtue of experience, without having undergone a recognised course and examinations system.

The term, *nurse practitioner*, originated in the United States. The first nurse practitioner in the UK, whose background was in health visiting, took up her post in Birmingham in 1982. Since then the numbers have grown considerably. Some nurse practitioners undertake work with neglected, underprivileged groups in the community; others work in hospitals, general practice or walk-in centres. Each nurse practitioner has to identify and establish his/her own sphere of influence. Nurse practitioners continue to wait for their own special skills and expertise to be recognised and protected by the UKCC because the issue has not been addressed satisfactorily[9]. Meanwhile, there can be an overlap with some of the work of practice nurses and the titles may still be used rather indiscriminately. Conflict can arise in a practice which employs a nurse practitioner and a practice nurse, both of whom have qualified at degree level and expect to be accorded the same level of respect. It is essential that a clear understanding is reached, so that the patients benefit from the expertise of all the nurses.

Skill-mix

Skill-mix is the name of the system for identifying the knowledge and expertise needed to perform any job, so that the most appropriate person can do it. Nurses in hospitals and the community have become accustomed to skill-mix reviews but it is relatively new to general practice[10]. Any nurse who wishes to review his/her role can consider each activity in turn and list the knowledge, skills and education needed to perform it effectively. It will become apparent which activities could be delegated to a health care assistant and a case can then be made on economic grounds for utilising nursing skills most effectively. Phlebotomy is a case in point, for while it can reasonably be argued that practice nurses may deal with other important issues while taking blood, it may be hard to justify the routine use of a highly trained nurse in such a role. The nurse practitioner and nurse triage roles could be considered as examples of skill-mix; using nursing and medical expertise most effectively.

Nurse employment in general practice

Medical training has traditionally been concerned with diagnosis and treatment, with little time left over for management and issues of human resources.

It follows that while some GPs are excellent employers, there are others who are less so. This can leave an inexperienced nurse vulnerable to exploitation. The terms and conditions agreed at the interview are binding, but employees are entitled to receive a written contract of employment within two months of starting work[11]. Part-time workers have the same rights as full-time staff. Employees rights were enhanced by new employment legislation in 1999, which established new rules for fair treatment of employees, the right to trade union representation and to family-friendly policies[12].

Nurses accustomed to pay and conditions negotiated nationally may have never had to negotiate on their own behalf before. Not all nurses are naturally assertive, so it is important to know what to ask at the interview and how to present a good case when negotiating for a change in conditions or salary. The RCN and other trade unions have produced guidelines on the employment of practice nurses. The following points should be considered in relation to employment.

Job description

A job description should specify the job title, the key activities and responsibilities, the conditions of employment, clinical grade and salary and to whom the employee is accountable. A comprehensive job description also provides a tool for appraisal at a performance review.

The RCN guidelines on employment for practice nurses specify the type of work and the responsibility suitable to each grade, although all NHS employees will undergo a regrading exercise in the near future and practice nurses are unlikely to be exempted[13].

Job descriptions can prevent misunderstandings if everyone involved knows what they are required to do. When all staff members have a job description, it will become apparent if the responsibility for those small tasks necessary to the smooth running of a practice has not been specified. Unnecessary conflict can be prevented if such issues are resolved promptly.

Contract of employment

A statement of terms of employment should cover the following:

- Salary and incremental dates; rates of pay for overtime hours
- The normal hours and times of work plus expectations of overtime to cover the absence of colleagues
- Holiday, study leave, sick pay, maternity/parental leave and compassionate leave entitlements
- Pension arrangements
- Period of notice at the termination of the employment.

In addition, the contract should set out the disciplinary and grievance procedures. Any health and safety hazards in the place of employment should also be included. If home visiting is part of the job description, then a mileage and car allowance should be negotiated. Practice nurses are strongly advised to seek a contract which guarantees pay and conditions of service in line with those of other NHS nurses.

Pensions

Pensions need careful consideration. Since 1997 practice employees have been entitled to contribute to the NHS pension scheme and to receive an employer's contribution. The practice manager will be able to provide advice on NHS pensions and any additional voluntary contributions which may be paid. Many people wait until middle age before considering pension arrangements but it is worth getting independent advice as soon as possible, about the best ways of maximising income after retirement.

Insurance

National Insurance contributions are deducted at source from the salary, together with contributions made by the employer, pay for sickness, maternity and unemployment benefit and for the state pension. GPs have indemnity insurance to cover vicarious liability for injury caused by their employees. However, personal indemnity insurance is essential because nurses, as individuals, could also be sued. The Royal College of Nursing, Medical Defence Union, the Community Practitioners and Health Visitors Association (CPHVA) and Unison provide indemnity insurance and give legal advice to members if needed.

Accountability

Accountability for one's actions is one of the hallmarks of a professional person. Ultimately nurses are accountable to their patients, via the UKCC, for the standards of nursing care provided. Among other things, the *Code of Professional Conduct* requires all nurses to refuse to accept delegated tasks for which they are not adequately trained[14]. Many aspects of practice nursing go far beyond what is taught pre-registration and nurses may sometimes feel pressurised to take on work for which they are not adequately prepared. Assertiveness training can be helpful in dealing with difficult situations, but it is up to every nurse to ensure that he she practices safely.

   The Scope of Professional Practice outlines the criteria for developing the nursing role[15]. It frees nurses from many previous petty restrictions and allows them to accept new challenges; providing all the UKCC guidelines for safeguarding the public are followed.

Professional registration

Current registration with the UKCC is required in order to practice as a nurse. The registration fee and notification of the intention to practice is sent every three years. Each registered nurse is issued with a plastic card, bearing a personal identification number (PIN). Evidence of professional updating and learning, needs to be available in a Personal Professional Profile as part of the requirements for reregistration. A minimum of five days study in three years must be undertaken in subjects relevant to the area of work. Many practice nurses already achieve much more than this, but arrangements are needed to help those who do not. Formal study days are not necessary, as long as the learning and its influence on nursing practice is documented[16].

The UKCC and four national boards were replaced by a new body – the Nurses and Midwives Council in April 2002, although concerns have been expressed about the way the new body will function[17]. The number of professional representatives has been drastically reduced.

Appraisal and professional development

It is expected nowadays, that staff will have a regular performance review, which should help to identify the strengths and weaknesses in their work, identify their learning needs and contribute to their professional development. All practitioners are expected to have a personal development plan and be able to demonstrate when their personal objectives have been met. Appraisal interviews should not be confused with disciplinary procedures.

Networking for support

Traditionally practice nurses have been thought to work in greater isolation than other groups of nurses and while this may be true in some instances, there is a large support network stretching out for those who look for it. The loss of public confidence in elements of the health service, as a result of various scandals in recent times, calls for all practitioners to be able to demonstrate their competence. The use of support networks is vital to achieve this aim.

Local support

Clinical supervision

Although not a new concept, clinical supervision was slow to develop among practice nurses because of their unique employment status, but is now being recognised as a valuable means of support and of promoting high standards. Various ways have been suggested for organising clinical supervision, either in groups or on a one-to-one basis and every nurse should be able to access the form of clinical supervision to suit him/herself[18].

Practice nurse groups

Local practice nurse groups developed spontaneously across the country as practice nursing developed, but as other educational and support opportunities arose, local groups sometimes became redundant. However there is still a need for groups of nurses to meet to share ideas and listen to speakers on topics of common interest. Nursing audit and quality control groups meet to consider aspects of nursing practice and standards of care.

Regional support

Some local practice nurse groups are affiliated to regional associations, which can often lobby for change more effectively than small groups and individuals. The National Practice Nurses Conference and Exhibition is planned and organised by a different regional group each year, either alone or in conjunction with other organisations such as the RCN. About 500 nurses attend the three-day event, which provides a chance for social contact with colleagues as well as topical lectures and seminars.

National support

The RCN Practice Nurse Association is active on behalf of its members and all the specialist groups within the RCN run study days and conferences. The Community Practitioners and Health Visitors' Association and Unison also offer membership to practice nurses.

The Internet is an ideal way for nurses to network. The Practice Nurse E-Group allows nurses to contact colleagues from any area in order to seek or provide information. The group has a facility for sharing protocols, and contributors often provide the web address of other useful Internet sites.

Practice nurse education

When the UKCC policy on community nurse education came into operation in 1996 (see Chapter 1), transitional arrangements were made for experienced practice nurses to acquire a recordable qualification in line with the automatic use of the title given to the district nurses and health visitors, who qualified under the previous system. Most areas have experienced practice nurses in post with teaching qualifications, who act as specialist practice teachers (SPTs). Training practices are also being designated, where a practice nurse who has qualified in teaching and assessing provides supervision and support for nurses in training. Since September 2001 a new system for educating nurse teachers has been instituted in response to the UKCC enquiry into nurse education. This was mainly concerned with pre-registration education, rather than preparation for specialist practice[19]. Mentors, practice educators and lecturers have become the only recordable nurse-teaching qualifications[20]. Education courses for community specialist practice teachers have been discontinued.

Practice development nurses

The valuable support of the primary care facilitator was lost in many areas as health authorities prepared to devolve responsibility to primary care organisations. Although some practice nurses were left in limbo for a time, the new primary care trusts have usually appointed practice development nurses with the inclusion of the interests of practice nurses in their roles. At the present time, few of these practice development nurses have a direct managerial responsibility for practice nurses but all professional staff are required to meet agreed standards of practice as a part of clinical governance. Workforce planning has a high priority in the new NHS[21]. It is a part of the practice development role and new nurses need to be attracted to practice nursing if a shortage is to be avoided in the future. Nurses who have had a career break may have to undertake a back-to-nursing course before returning to practice. Distance learning can be particularly suited to practice nurses, many of whom work part time. There has been a rapid increase in the number and type of courses and modules available.

Journals

A wide variety of nursing journals is available. *Practice Nurse* and *Practice Nursing* are written specifically for practice nurses. Other journals such as *Community Nurse* and *Primary Health Care* are published for all community nurses, while *Nursing Times* and *Nursing Standard* are examples of journals of interest to all branches of nursing. *Evidence-Based Nursing* and *The Journal of Advanced Nursing* publish nursing research findings to help inform evidence-based practice. Journals provide much more up-to-date material than textbooks and every nurse should read the journals most relevant to his/her work. Many practices will purchase the journals needed by clinical staff to keep up to date.

CATS, APEL and APL

Credit accumulation and transfer (CATS) is a way of evaluating the academic content of different courses so that points can be collected towards an academic award. Three levels of credit are awarded in England and Wales:

(1)   120 credits at level 1 = certificate level
(2)   + 120 credits at level 2 = diploma level
(3)   + 120 credits at level 3 = degree level
      Scotland has four levels of credits (SCOTCATS).

Assessment of prior experiential learning (APEL) is a way of awarding credits for previous learning. Life experiences, professional knowledge and skills are assessed and credited towards a relevant academic course. A professional profile needs to be prepared, which outlines previous learning experiences and the ways they have influenced practice. Colleges usually charge for these assessments, which are complex to administer.

Assessment of prior learning (APL) allows credits to be awarded for relevant courses and examination results.

Identifying good practice

Reflection

All nurses are expected to make time to reflect on situations in their own practice and to learn from both positive outcomes and those which could have been handled differently[22]. Reflections on practice can also be an essential part of clinical supervision sessions and written reflections form part of the professional profile to demonstrate learning from experience.

Evidence-based practice

Increased public expectations and the growth of communications mean that practitioners must be able to base their practice on the best available evidence. Since no doctor or nurse could possibly read and consider all the material relevant to his/her sphere of work, ways are needed to assess the validity of evidence and disseminate information on best practice. The National Institute for Clinical Excellence was established to make recommendations and distribute guidelines on clinical treatments. The Internet allows access to a wealth of material, although discrimination is required because anyone can post information on the net; not all of it is reliable. The RCN Research and Development Coordinating Centre runs a database providing direct links to many useful sources and databases of systematic reviews. Local clinical librarians will usually help anyone who needs assistance to search for evidence. The NHS Health Technology Assessment Programme has information dissemination systems which include:

- The UK Cochrane Centre and Library
- NHS centre for Reviews and Dissemination, York
- NHS Research and Development Projects Register.

Despite the wealth of information available, some nursing practice has still not changed significantly in response to research findings and there has been a conspicuous lack of good research in the field of practice nursing. The clinical governance agenda makes it imperative for practitioners to establish strong theoretical foundations to their practice in order to give good clinical care.

Audit

Audit means measuring what is actually being done; compared with an agreed standard of practice. For example, a practice could have a policy for all diabetic patients to be reviewed annually, i.e. 100% of diabetic patients. Taking an audit would involve looking at the records of all patients with diabetes to see when they were last reviewed. As an example, it might transpire that only 85% of the patients were reviewed in the past year.

There is no point in doing this exercise unless the practice is prepared to act on the findings and take steps to remedy the deficiencies, but having done so, the audit should be repeated to see if the percentage rate has improved. The use of computers can make audit a less onerous task – providing the data being sought has actually been entered. In many instances, written records still have to be retrieved and examined. This whole process is known as the audit cycle:

- Select a suitable topic which is measurable, has definable standards and is amenable to change
- Agree the standard for best practice
- Collect the information
- Compare the information with the standard
- Plan any changes needed
- Implement the changes
- Re-audit to see if improvements have been made.

Local primary care audit advisory groups welcome nurse involvement in audit and will usually provide helpful advice and training. Nurses are also employed by some organisations and drug companies to advise on nursing and medical audit.

Nursing research

Research explores the boundaries and establishes the body of knowledge required to practice in a profession. Research may be an academic and exhaustive study based in a university department but it can simply be the questioning of routine procedures or asking the question 'why' in relation to day-to-day work. A practice nurse could be involved with research in several ways:

- Keeping his/her own knowledge up to date by reading research reports, or conducting a literature search on a particular topic
- Designing a study to test an idea for improving nursing practice
- Taking part in a wider research programme organised by a general practitioner, research nurse, or other outside body.

The term *hierarchy of evidence* is commonly used in relation to research, with greater credence being given to the methods considered to be most rigorous and providing the strongest evidence[23].

Quantitative studies[24]

Prospective randomised controlled trials (RCTs) are considered to provide the best evidence about the effectiveness of healthcare interventions. Participants are randomly allocated to either an experimental group or a control group. Since all the characteristics of both groups are meant to be the same, any difference in outcome should be due to the intervention. Some of the problems of RCTs include:

- Difficulties with randomisation
- Ethical issues when using a placebo or withholding a potentially valuable treatment
- Cost
- The length of time before the outcome of the trial is known
- Generalisability – can the results of the trial be transferred to people other than those studied?

Many nursing activities, by their very nature, do not lend themselves readily to RCTs.

Cohort studies identify and measure exposure to a risk or treatment. Intervention and control groups are used and the outcomes analysed. The lack of randomisation can mean that results could be due to variations between the groups unrelated to the intervention being studied.

Case control studies are used retrospectively to compare one group with a particular condition to a similar group without the condition, in order to compare exposure to the risk factor by both groups and thus to establish a causal relationship.

Qualitative studies

Qualitative studies often attempt to explain what is happening in a given situation. Observation and interviews are commonly used methods for this type of research. The aim is to increase understanding of those particular situations. Therefore, sampling in this type of research is not randomised from the whole population but from the people likely to have the experiences being studied. Qualitative reports often contain direct quotes from participants to illustrate the study theme[25]. Much of the research into nursing tends to be quantitative in nature.

Systematic reviews

Various groups have evolved to help practitioners to make decisions based on the best available evidence. Systematic reviews rigorously assess the research evidence available. The various databases provide information about reviews completed and in progress.

Suggestions for reflection on practice

- Analyse your job description. Are there any activities which could be delegated? Are there any activities for which you need more education or supervision?
- Does your professional profile provide a comprehensive account of your learning? What are your professional development goals?
- How would you know if your nursing practice could be improved?

Further reading

Bishop, V. & Scott, I. (eds) (2001) *Challenges in Clinical Practice. Professional developments in nursing.* Palgrave, Basingstoke.

Carey, L. (2000) *Practice Nursing.* Bailliere Tindall in association with the Royal College of Nursing, London.

Cook, R. (1999) *A Nurse's Survival Guide to Primary Care.* Churchill Livingstone, Edinburgh.

Distance Learning, *Healthcare Assistants Programme – Parts 1, 2 and 3.* Radcliffe, Oxford.

Jarvis, S. (2001) Skill mix in primary care – implications for the future. Medical Practices Committee, *www.doh.gov.uk/pdfs/skillmix.pdf* (accessed 10/9/01).

Royal College of Nursing (1997) *Nurse Practitioners – your questions answered.* Royal College of Nursing, London.

Spouse, J. & Redfern, L. (eds) (2000) *Successful Supervision in Health Care Practice.* Blackwell Science, Oxford.

Taylor, B. (2000) *Reflective Practice.* Open University Press, Buckingham.

References

1. Royal College of Nursing (1998) *Clinical Governance: guidance for nurses.* RCN, London.
2. Atkin, K., Lunt, N., Parker, G. & Hurst, M. (1993) *Nurses Count: a national census of practice nurses.* Social Policy Research Unit, University of York.
3. DHSS (1986) *Neighbourhood Nursing – a Focus for Care.* HMSO, London.
4. Woolnough, F. (1990) A crisis of identity. *Practice Nurse*, **2**, 447–8, 454.
5. Audit Commission (1993) *Practice Makes Perfect: the Role of the Family Health Service Authorities.* HMSO, London.

6. United Kingdom Central Council for Nurses, Midwives and Health Visitors (1986) *Project 2000: a New Preparation for Practice*. UKCC, London.
7. The Centre for Innovation in Primary Care (2000) *What do practice nurses do? A study of roles, responsibilities and patterns of work*. The Centre for Innovation in Primary Care, Sheffield.
8. Macdougald, N., King, P., Jones, A. & Everleigh, M. (2000) *A Toolkit for Practice Nurses*. Aeneas Press, Chichester.
9. Chamber, N. (1998) *Nurse Practitioners in Primary Care*. Radcliffe Medical Press, Oxford.
10. Royal College of Nursing (1992) *Skill Mix and Reprofiling: a guide for RCN members*, Royal College of Nursing, London.
11. Royal College of Nursing (2000) *Guidance on Employing Nurses in General Practice*. Royal College of Nursing, London.
12. Parliament (1999) *The Employment Relations Act* 1999 HMSO, London.
13. Department of Health (1998) *Agenda for Change – Modernising the NHS Pay System*. Department of Health, London.
14. UKCC (1992) *Code of Professional Conduct*. Para. 4. UKCC, London.
15. UKCC (1992) *The Scope of Professional Practice*. UKCC, London.
16. UKCC (2001) *The PREP Handbook*. UKCC, London.
17. Norman, A. (2001) *The Future of Professional Regulation – the UKCC's response. Register. Number 36*. UKCC, London.
18. UKCC (2001) *Supporting Nurses, Midwives and Health Visitors through Lifelong Learning*, p. 6. UKCC, London.
19. Peach, L. (Chair) (1999) The UKCC Commission for Nursing and Midwifery Education. *Fitness for Practice*. UKCC, London.
20. UKCC (2000) *Standards for the Preparation of Teachers of Nursing, Midwifery and Health Visiting*. UKCC, London.
21. Department of Health (2000) *A Health Service of all the Talents: Developing the NHS workforce*. HMSO, London.
22. Freshwater, D. (1998) *Transforming Nursing through Reflective Practice*. Blackwell Science, Oxford.
23. Author unknown (February 1995) Evidence and effectiveness, *Bandolier*, 12: *www.bandolier.net/band12/bd12* (accessed 12/9/01).
24. Roberts, J. & DiCenso, A. (1999) Identifying the best research design to fit the question. Part 1. *Evidence-Based Nursing*, **2** (1), 4–6.
25. Ploeg, J. (1999) Identifying the best research design to fit the question. Part 2. *Evidence-Based Nursing*, **2** (2), 36–7.

Useful addresses and web sites

Community Practitioners' and Health Visitors' Association
40 Bermondsey Street, London SE1 3UD
Telephone: 020 7939 7000 Fax: 020 7403 2976
Web site: *www.msfcphva.org.uk*

Medical Defence Union
230 Blackfriars Road, London SE1 8PJ
Telephone: 020 7202 1500 *Fax:* 020 7202 1666
Web site: *www.the-mdu.com*

Open University
PO Box 625, Milton Keynes MK7 6YG
Web site: *www.open.ac.uk*

Practice Nursing
Mark Allen Publishing Ltd, Croxted Mews, 286a–288 Croxted Rd, London SE24 9BY
Subscription – Freephone: 0800 137 201

Practice Nurse subscriptions
Freepost RCC2619, Haywards Heath, West Sussex RH16 3BR

Royal College of Nursing
20 Cavendish Square, London W1G 0RN
Telephone: 020 7409 3333
Web site: *www.rcn.org.uk*

RCN Direct
24 hour information and advice for members of RCN
Telephone: 0845 7726100

United Kingdom Central Council for Nurses, Midwives and Health Visitors
23 Portland Place, London WIN 3AF
Telephone: 020 7637 7181 Fax: 020 7436 2924
Web site: *www.ukcc.org.uk*

Electronic mail

Practice Nurse E-Group
http://groups.yahoo.com/groups/practicenurse

Web sites

NHS Centre for Reviews and Dissemination, University of York.
www.york.ac.uk

NHS R & D Health Technology Assessment Programme
www.hta.nhsweb.nhs.uk

RCN Research & Development Coordination Centre
www.man.ac.uk/rcn/d&udatabase.htm

UK Department of Health Research – National Research Register
www.doh.gov.uk/research

Chapter 3
Practice Organisation

Information about patients

The staff in general practice have access to a great deal of information, which raises important issues about the way that information is utilised and stored.

Confidentiality

Patients have a right to expect that any personal information about them will remain confidential. The confidential aspects of the work must be impressed on all staff members when they join the practice and the consequence of breaching confidentiality must be made explicit in the statement of terms of employment.

The UKCC Code of Professional Conduct insists that nurses may only disclose confidential information: if the patient gives consent, if a court order is served or if the wider public interest justifies the disclosure[1]. Unwitting breaches can occur unless careful steps are taken to prevent them. There are risks to confidentiality in any of the following situations:

- Conversations or telephone calls in the hearing of other patients
- Discussing a patient with a third party without consent
- Gossip about incidents which occur at work
- Computer screens which show other patients' details
- Records left lying open
- Personal information in the rubbish bin.

Computers with a screen saver facility will stop showing data after a few minutes but it is much better to get into the habit of clearing the screen immediately after use. Apart from heightened staff awareness, thought given to the design of reception and waiting areas and to soundproofing consulting rooms, can prevent conversations from being overheard. Manual records must be filed as soon as possible and computer systems must be secure. Any waste paper which could identify patients needs to be shredded. Investigation results must not be given to anyone other than the person who had the test, unless they have given their consent to disclosure. As a cautionary tale, picture the effect on the wife who was told by a receptionist that her husband's post-vasectomy sperm count was negative, when as it turned out, the wife herself had already had a sterilisation operation!

There should be a practice policy to cover situations when a patient does not speak English. An interpreter, who is not a family member of the patient, should be arranged whenever possible. Link workers are able to interpret and act as advocates in areas with mixed ethnic populations. We live in a multi-cultural society and although lip-service is paid to this fact, many nurses have not been taught how to meet the health needs of people from different back-grounds. Training in cultural awareness is provided locally for health and social care workers. All practice nurses are advised to access this training.

Record systems

A good record system is vital for the efficient management of patient care. Practice nurses are major contributors to the information system and to this end it is important to understand the records systems. The purpose of a record is:

- To record all the relevant information about a patient
- To enable appropriate preventive care to be offered to patients
- To facilitate the management of patients with chronic diseases
- To enable all members of the PHCT to work together for the benefit of the patients
- To act as a focus for the education of GP registrars and other members of the PHCT
- To enable data to be extracted for practice audit, performance review and research purposes
- To provide evidence, if required, for medico-legal purposes.

The medical record envelope

The medical record envelopes, still known as 'Lloyd George envelopes', have been the main source of information about patients since they were introduced in 1911; the year that Lloyd George started a national health insurance scheme for working men. The fact that the envelopes have been around for so long says something for their durability but also explains why, in the twenty-first cen-tury, their size may be inadequate for a lifetime's health record.

The continuation cards in the record should be in chronological order and tagged together. Letters should be trimmed to fit in the envelope easily. Letters and test results should also be tagged separately in chronological order. Besides this simple and very basic record there are a number of insert cards which can be obtained to expand the information available.

Summary card The summary card (contrarily pink for males and blue for females) is used to summarise all the important details about a patient. Inclusion of a summary card is a requirement for training practices in many parts of the country, although much of this information is now held on computer instead.

Immunisation record cards   Immunisation record cards allow all the routine and travel vaccines given to be seen at a glance. This makes it easier to see when immunisations have been missed or reinforcing doses are due.

A4 records

Mention has already been made of the small size of the 'Lloyd George envelopes'. Since the 1970s a number of practices have adopted A4 (297 × 210 cm) records, the standard size for hospital notes. Fund-holding generated a great deal of extra correspondence, which in turn caused storage problems and an expansion of medical records.

Computers

Computerised record systems in general practice are now commonplace. Many practices still use manual records as well but more practices are becoming 'paperlight'; relying more and more on computers. A plan of action should be prepared in case of a computer failure and all the users have a responsibility to protect the system as much a possible. Apart from the obvious uses, such as recording registration information, clinical notes and printing prescriptions, computers can be used for many other purposes:

- Computerised appointment systems allow information to be gathered easily about waiting times, length of consultations and non-attendance. Doctors and nurses can also see on screen which patients have arrived.

- Disease registers can be accessed quickly (providing the data has been recorded on the computer in the first place).

- Searches can be made for a variety of reasons:
  - Call and recall of patients with specific medical conditions, e.g. asthma, diabetes, hypertension, or for health promotion, e.g. children for immunisation, women due for cervical smears, patients aged over 65 for flu injections. Mail merge can be used to produce standard call/recall letters.
  - Patients receiving a particular medication can be identified for research purposes, audit or drug checks.

- Databases of useful information can be kept such as voluntary services and self-help groups. There are electronic versions of familiar books such as the *BNF* and *MIMS*. Some clinical systems also provide patient information leaflets.

- The Internet provides a gateway to a world of information. Travel health is just one area about which practice nurses might want to seek information.

- The NHSNet is a national, virtually private network, used by hospitals, health authorities, GP practices and others. It is protected from unauthorised access via the Internet by firewalls and other security devices. As electronic recording and messaging becomes more and more part of the way people work in the NHS, this network will be carrying increasing volumes of information.

At present, electronic links allow registration data and item of service claims to be sent directly to the health authority, and pathology results to be received from the laboratory. Over time, practices will be able to send test requests and receive more information, such as discharge summaries and x-ray results from hospitals via the NHSNet. The transmission of pictures, for such specialties as dermatology, is being used successfully in more rural areas for remote consultations with hospital consultants.

Although computers are exciting to use, there are security, reliability and confidentiality aspects to be considered as well:

- A plan of action should be prepared in case of a computer failure and all users have a responsibility to protect the system as much as possible.

- A modem and service provider allows access to the Internet. However, a modem also renders a computer system vulnerable to hackers, who can invade a system for fun or to access patient information. Entry to the system should be protected by codes and passwords, which must be unique to each user, changed regularly and kept as secret as any cash card personal identification number.

- Under the terms of the Data Protection Act computer users have to be registered as data users[2]. This is usually arranged by the practice manager.

- Every practice should have one person, preferably a health professional, responsible for computer security. This person is known as a Caldicott guardian[3].

- The machines are only as good as the people who write the programmes and every system has some limitations. A fault in the programme (bug) can lead to some bizarre results at times.

- A power failure or a fault with the equipment could cause essential patient information to be lost. For this reason daily copies of all the data must be made and a copy of this back-up kept off site in case of fire or theft in the practice.

- All staff have a responsibility for the security of the building. Procedures for locking windows and doors must be followed rigorously. Computer equipment can be very attractive to burglars and the loss of both the hardware and the data could be devastating.

The facilities and health protection required for staff who work with visual display units (VDUs) are laid down in Health and Safety Executive regulations[4].

Disease register

A register of patients with specific conditions can be compiled, using a computer or a card system by all of the following means:

- At registration, during registration health checks
- When diagnosed in the practice or a letter is received from a hospital
- During consultations, when being seen for another reason
- From repeat prescriptions.

Disease registers have assumed an even greater importance since the introduction of national service frameworks and health improvement programmes, because practices need to be able to audit the care of specific groups of patients.

Practices are also required to compile a register of all their patients who are carers, even if the person for whom they care is not registered with that practice[5].

Access to records

In the past, medical records were jealously guarded from the eyes of the people most concerned – the patients themselves. As a result of which, sardonic comments in the notes, such as 'this patient enjoys very poor health,' were not uncommon. Patients were not told the whole truth about their illness, especially if the prognosis was poor. Alternatively, if the records later became mislaid, a patient might never learn what the original diagnosis had been.

The attitude to disclosure is now quite different and most patients expect to be given factual information. In the main, patients have a legal right to see any information held about them in computer files[6]. A formal request in writing should be made. The doctor then has up to 40 days to provide the information, together with an explanation of any technical codes or abbreviations. Since 1 November 1991 patients have also had a right of access to written records made after that date. The records of all health professionals, including nurses, are covered by the Access to Health Records Act (1990). A doctor can refuse to disclose information held manually or on computer in the following circumstances:

- If he/she considers that serious mental or physical harm could be caused as a result
- To protect the confidentiality of a third party who might be identified from the patients' records.

Nurses' own records

Most nurses write directly into the patients' NHS or computer records. Nursing records should provide a comprehensive, chronological account which covers:

- An assessment of the patients general health and the specific problems identified
- The type of care planned
- The nursing interventions, advice or information given
- The outcomes of the care given, and further actions planned or implemented.

In some instances, such as complicated wound care or travel immunisation, separate nursing records can be more appropriate; especially where two or more part-time nurses are treating the same patient. Good communication is essential for continuity of care. Nursing records, if they are separate, should be amalgamated with the patients' medical notes as soon as possible. In the event of litigation, records will be used to prove or disprove a case of negligence. Without accurate records, it would not be possible to prove that satisfactory care had been given.

The guidelines for record keeping issued by the UKCC clearly specify the nurse's responsibilities with regard to records[7]. Records should:

- Be factual and accurate, without using jargon or offensive statements, detailing the care and information given
- Be written as near as possible to the time of the consultation
- Be clearly, indelibly written and able to be photocopied
- Include the date, time and signature at each entry
- Show the original entry if any alteration is made; alterations or additions should be signed and dated.

Private patients

Many practices are designated Yellow Fever Centres, providing immunisation for patients who are not registered with the practice. People ineligible for NHS treatment may also be seen privately. There is no official record for private patients (unlike those for registered patients and temporary residents), but if injections or treatments are given privately, then a system must be in place for recording the relevant information for each patient.

Protocols, guidelines and clinical pathways

When a nurse joins a practice he/she will need to discuss the nursing role with colleagues. The exact scope and responsibility of each nurse will be governed by his/her previous experience and training. The limits of a nurse's freedom to act autonomously can be negotiated and then recorded in a protocol.

Protocols

This word *protocol* is used rather freely and can be viewed as either a protection or a threat. If a protocol is too rigid then any deviation from it could possibly place a practitioner at risk of prosecution if anything should go wrong. This is a particular concern of doctors, who fear being constrained to provide medical treatment exactly as specified in a treatment protocol[8]. On the other hand, many nurses feel they can work with greater confidence if they have agreed boundaries. Protocols tend to be prescriptive – outlining the actions required in a particular situation and the information to be given. Nurse-run clinics often follow a protocol. Computerised protocols are used by NHS Direct nurses to deal with telephone consultations and it is possible that practice nurses will soon use these same protocols to triage requests for urgent GP appointments[9]. Legislation has allowed for patient group directions to replace protocols for the administration of vaccines and drugs without prescription[10] (see Chapter 8, Common Medical Conditions).

Guidelines

Guidelines are generally considered to be less rigid than protocols and the term has become more commonly used. Systematic reviews and guidelines are regularly produced by the National Institute for Clinical Excellence. National and European bodies such as the British Thoracic Society and European Resuscitation Council produce guidelines in their respective fields of expertise. *Guidelines*, published in book form three times a year, provides up-to-date clinical guidelines for primary care.

Clinical pathways

A more recent addition to the terminology is *clinical pathways*. These are intended to be used by all members of the multidisciplinary team in primary and secondary care as a template for the coordination of treatment and care of patients with specific conditions. Clinical pathways meet the requirements of the new NHS to provide seamless care, with efficiency, effectiveness and involvement of the public[11]. Clinical pathways tend to have a locality focus, such as a *stroke pathway* used by everyone in a hospital and the community in a particular area. Whatever the terminology used, any protocol, guideline or clinical pathway must be reviewed regularly and updated in the light of new clinical evidence.

Policies and procedures

Policies or rules are needed in any organisation so that all the staff know what is expected of them. Some policies in general practice are dictated by legal statute or public safety requirements. For example:

- Health and safety issues, in accordance with the Health and Safety at Work directives

- Manual handling
- Fire regulations, covering the maintenance of fire extinguishers, staff training, and the procedure in the event of a fire
- Control of infection, covering the handling of specimens, dealing with body fluids, the disposal of sharps and clinical waste, methods of preventing cross-infection.

Other policies may cover more domestic issues such as: the arrangement of holidays and study leave, communicating messages, setting healthy examples for the public, avoiding waste of energy and resources.

Complaints

If there is dissatisfaction with any aspect of treatment, the problem may be resolved amicably, by discussion, in preference to a formal complaint. Where a policy of openness already exists, patients may have no need to resort to the law. However, since 1996 all practices have been required to have a formal policy for dealing with complaints[12]. In the first instance this may be to the practice manager or senior partner, but patients and the staff must be made aware of the practice complaints procedure.

Appointments

Practices have different ways of arranging access for patients to the GP or practice nurse. With a simple queuing system patients arrive at the beginning of surgery and are seen on a first-come, first-served basis. This can lead to long waits for patients and a lack of control by practitioners over their consulting time.

Appointment systems allow the workload to be spaced out and planned in advance, which in theory should save patients from having to wait more than a few minutes to be seen. However, patients cannot be ill by appointment, so time must always be set aside for dealing with urgent problems. If an emergency arises during surgery time, the booked appointments are likely to be delayed. Most people will accept such delays providing they are kept informed and do not feel they are being treated unfairly. Computerised appointment systems can log the time a patient arrived, when the patient was seen, and even how long the consultation took – all valuable information for auditing the effectiveness of the organisation. Even without a computer, audits can be conducted to identify ways of improving the system.

If patients do not keep their appointments, this is not only a waste of professional time, it can also deprive other patients of the chance to be seen sooner. A graph in the waiting area, showing the number of hours wasted by non-attenders each week, can remind the public about their responsibilities towards the service.

Practice nurses who use appointment systems can give the receptionists a list of the times to be allowed for specific procedures and consultations. A policy of allowing patients to select times to suit themselves can increase the number of people who are able to attend for health promotion and screening.

Investigation results

A system is needed for ensuring that patients get the results of investigations. A patient must either know when to return to the surgery or when to telephone for results. Abnormal results should not be filed until the necessary steps have been taken for the patient to be followed up.

Telephone calls

A policy is needed for the handling of telephone calls. Too many interruptions during surgery time can be disruptive but patients have to be put through in urgent situations. Other callers can be given a time to call back; although no patient should have to ring more than twice. Some doctors and nurses overcome this problem by having allotted telephone times for giving test results, or dealing with other enquiries. Any advice given over the telephone should be recorded in the patient's records, and telephone messages should be written down immediately in case they get forgotten. A record must be kept of all visit requests. It is now possible to use a computerised system to record all incoming and outgoing telephone calls from a practice. This is not illegal but nurses are advised to ensure that patients are aware that calls are being recorded, in case they choose not to discuss confidential issues on the telephone.

Meetings

Clinical meetings between members of the primary health care team are essential for exchanging information and giving feedback about patients, as well as providing learning opportunities for all concerned. Support can also be offered to individual team members who are dealing with stressful situations.

Joint staff meetings are valuable when domestic policies are being decided. Compliance will be better if everyone has been consulted and understands the need for the policy. Off-the-cuff pronouncements, which are subsequently changed, can be very damaging for morale. Team meetings need to be structured so that everyone is able to make a valid contribution and when decisions are reached, everyone who is likely to be affected must be made aware of them.

Social gatherings, like a Christmas party or summer barbecue, can cement good relationships within the team. The more that people meet together informally as well as formally, the better they will understand and support each other.

Public involvement

Involvement of patients is a key part of the NHS reforms. Some practices and health centres already have valuable consumer groups, where patient representatives can make suggestions or take practical steps for improving the service. Some patient groups are highly organised with fund-raising committees and groups to support the housebound, bereaved patients or mothers with young children. Patient satisfaction questionnaires are frequently used to obtain the views of patients about primary care services. Care is needed in developing a suitable questionnaire so that the purpose of the survey is made clear, it is unambiguous and patient anonymity is preserved[13]. Information about age, gender, ethnicity and occupation should also be requested in case any of these variables have a bearing on the responses to the questions.

Suggestions for reflection on practice

- How easy is it to maintain confidentiality in your working area? How could any improvements be made?
- Are you using your computer system fully? What further training is needed?
- Does all your record-keeping meet the UKCC standards?
- Are the protocols/guidelines you use evidence-based? Are they due for review?
- How much are the patients involved in your practice? Could more be done to encourage public involvement?

Further reading

Health and Safety Executive (1999) Health and safety in small firms. *An Introduction to Health and Safety.* Health and Safety Executive Books, Suffolk.

Holland, K. & Hogg, C. (2001) *Cultural Awareness in Nursing and Healthcare: An introductory text.* Arnold, London.

References

1. United Kingdom Central Council for Nurses, Midwives and Health Visitors (1992) *Code of Professional Conduct.* Para. 10, UKCC, London.
2. Parliament (1998) *Data Protection Act 1998.* HMSO, London.
3. NHS Executive (1997) *The Caldicott Committee: Report on the review of patient-identifiable information.* HMSO, London.
4. Health and Safety Executive (1992) *Display Screen Equipment Work – Guidance on*

Health and Safety (Display Screen Equipment) Regulations. Health and Safety Executive, Sheffield.

5. Department of Health (1999) *Caring About Carers: a national strategy for carers.* HMSO, London.
6. Parliament (1990) *Access to Health Records Act 1990.* HMSO, London.
7. United Kingdom Central Council for Nurses, Midwives and Health Visitors (1998) *Guidelines for Records and Record Keeping.* UKCC, London.
8. Pitts, J. (1993) Protocols for acute conditions. *Update,* **47** (12), 785–6.
9. Robinson, J. (2001) GPs working patterns set for shake-up. *Pulse,* **61** (34), 1.
10. Statutory Instrument (2000) *The Prescription only Medicines (Human Use) amended order, 2000.* Statutory Instrument No. 1917. HMSO, London.
11. National Assembly for Wales (2001) Health. *Clinical Pathways. www.wales.gov.uk/subihealth/content/keypubs/clinical* (accessed 3/9/01).
12. Statutory Instrument No. 669 (1996) *NHS England and Wales: The National Health Service (Function of Health Authorities) (Complaints) Regulations 1996.* Department of Health, London.
13. Collins, K. (1999) Developing patient satisfaction questionnaires. *Nursing Standard.* **14** (11), 37–8.

Useful addresses and web sites

Health and Safety Executive Information Centre
Broad Lane, Sheffield S3 7HG
Infoline Telephone: 08701 545500
Web site *www.open.gov.uk/hse/hsehome.htm*

National Association for Patient Participation (NAPP)
PO Box 999, Nuneaton, Warks CV11 5DZ
Telephone/Fax: 01051 630 5786
Web site: *www.napp.org.uk*

Web sites

Complaints procedures for the Department of Health *www.doh.gov.uk/complain.htm*

Chapter 4
Management of the Nurses' Rooms

As the work in general practice and the number of nurses increases, the accommodation needed by the practice nurses can change. The basic requirements include:

- A treatment/consulting room
- A waiting area for patients
- An accessible toilet for patients to use, including wheelchair access
- A secure storeroom
- A safe area for storing clinical waste and sharps before collection
- Access to a changing room and refreshment area or common room.

The practice nurse(s) should be involved when new or extended buildings are planned. The extra rooms or refinements to the nurses' accommodation might then include:

- A separate consulting room
- A separate minor surgery room
- An annexe to the treatment room for dealing with used instruments and specimens etc.
- Office space for administration
- A non-clinical room for counselling
- A room for group sessions.

The Disability Discrimination Act requires all buildings open to the public to meet designated standards of accessibility for the public and staff[1]. These regulations supersede the recommendations on premises in the *Statement of Fees and Allowances to General Practitioners* (the Red Book). Some premises might never be able to meet these stringent standards, so nurses could become involved in a move to new premises. NHS guidelines on designing new premises have been published[2]. There are also health and safety requirements on heating, ventilation, lighting and other aspects of the workplace, to be considered when designing a working environment[3].

Design and furnishing

A friendly environment can be created by the imaginative use of space and colour. Suitable storage space is needed to reduce clutter. Leaflet racks on the walls make information easily accessible, and pinboards are better than adhesive tape for displaying travel charts and other reference material. Attractive decor will create a welcoming atmosphere. Many people are nervous in a clinical environment: pictures, plants, and toys for children can help to put them at ease. Toys must be regularly washed with hot, soapy water and a routine check made to dispose of any broken or heavily contaminated toys. Concerns have been expressed about the risk of cross-infection from children's toys[4]. Nurses should be aware of the potential risk and follow the practice policy regarding the use of toys. Well-kept notice boards dealing with seasonal topics can have more impact than walls smothered with depressing posters condemning every known human weakness.

Lighting should be chosen with care. Bright, even lighting is needed in treatment areas and, in addition, directable lamps with heat filters are needed for minor surgery and cervical smears. Lamps must be easily cleanable. Softer lighting from lamps or wall lights is desirable for counselling or teaching relaxation. Blinds can be used to control sunlight and to provide privacy when needed. Basic furnishings include a desk, chairs, couch, lockable cupboards, and bookshelves. A curtained area or screen gives extra privacy and a mirror is helpful for the patients when they are getting dressed.

Treatment and minor surgery couches should be easily accessible, their covering non-permeable, and ideally, be height-adjustable. A secure step is needed for patients to get onto a non-adjustable couch. Patients will feel less intimidated if sitting at the same level as the nurse at the side of the desk, not being confronted across it. Comfortable chairs away from the desk are preferable for counselling and informal discussions. Furniture should be arranged so that the nurse's exit is not obstructed if a patient becomes aggressive. An alarm is needed for summoning help in any sort of emergency. Work surfaces and flooring in treatment areas should be hard-wearing, easy to clean and able to withstand bleach (in case of blood-spillage). A separate basin is needed for hand washing and a different, deep sink for washing used instruments. Both ought to have elbow taps and minimise splashing. There should be a dirty work area designated for dealing with specimens etc. All emergency equipment must be easily accessible. A visible plan of the location of all the equipment stored can save a nurse from returning to a scene of devastation after a day off!

Health and safety

Although work areas are planned for practicality, the overwhelming consideration should be for the safety of the public and staff. Employers are legally required to produce a safety policy and to report serious incidents to the Health and Safety Executive (HSE). All employees have a duty to take reasonable care to avoid injury to themselves or others and to cooperate with employers in meeting the statutory requirements for Health and Safety[5]. Manual handling training is a requirement for all staff[6].

Control of Substances Hazardous to Health (COSHH)

Employers are required to carry out a risk assessment for any substance which could be hazardous to health[7]. The assessment should cover:

- The name of the substance
- The type of hazard and precautions to be taken
- The planned use of the substance
- Possible unplanned events and the action to be taken.

Any staff member likely to be exposed to substances hazardous to health must understand the risks and the precautions to be taken to protect themselves and the public. Hazardous substances which might be used in general practice include: ethyl chloride, phenol, formaldehyde, potassium permanganate, silver nitrate, industrial spirit, sodium hypochlorite solution, liquid nitrogen, latex gloves, and contaminated waste.

Special precautions are needed if a mercury sphygmomanometer is broken because mercury is toxic. The mercury should be contained within the apparatus if possible, or be tipped into an airtight container, covered with water, and sealed. Mercury spillage kits are available, with special absorbent sponges and containers for storing the mercury for disposal. Detector pads left in the vicinity of the spillage will change colour if mercury fumes are present. The kits can be purchased, although they are relatively expensive. The handling of mercury waste is covered by COSHH regulations but mercury spillage counts as special waste and as such is subject to regulation under the Environment Protection Act (1990); it should not be put with clinical waste for incineration. Mercury sphygmomanometers are due to be phased out within a few years because of the risk to health and the environment from spilled mercury. Arrangements, probably for all PCT, will need to made for their safe disposal. Any new automated devices purchased should meet the recommendations of the British Hypertension Society for having the greatest agreement with mercury standards[8].

The storage of medicines and other substances

Controlled drugs are regulated under the Misuse of Drugs Act (1971). They must be stored in a special locked cupboard which is out of sight of windows and the public. A register must be kept on the premises for recording any new stock, the date it was obtained and the dispensing of any of the stock to patients or to individual doctors for their emergency bags. Out-of-date or unwanted controlled drugs may only be destroyed by persons authorised under the Misuse of Drugs Regulations, 1985[9].

Care must be taken with all drugs, lotions, vaccines and cleaning materials. They should always be kept in locked cupboards but because on occasions in a busy treatment room, a cupboard might accidentally be left unlocked, extra precautions are also sensible:

- All liquids should have childproof bottle tops and be stored out of reach of children. (The case of the unfortunate child who once gained access to a treatment room and drank some phenol, proved the need for such precautions[10].)
- Safety catches on cupboard doors and fridges will help to deter inquisitive toddlers.
- All trolleys must be cleared after use. (Imagine the effect of a silver nitrate pencil used as a play lipstick.)

The storage of vaccines

A doctor or nurse could be held liable for vaccination failure as a result of inadequate storage if it could be shown that the cold chain was intact before the product reached the practice. Vaccines must be stored at the temperatures specified by the manufacturers – usually between 2 and 8°C. Special vaccine fridges have a thermostatically controlled temperature range and a built-in maximum and minimum thermometer and alarm. This is the ideal way of storing vaccines but, whatever the type of fridge, it must be dedicated to vaccine storage alone and have a maximum/minimum thermometer for continuous temperature monitoring. A digital thermometer has a probe attached to a wire and can be used to map the coldest areas of the fridge. The display part of the digital thermometer can be fixed to the wall outside the fridge, so that the temperature can be seen at all times. The flexible wire passing into the fridge will not affect the door closure.

Some vaccines may have to be destroyed if the cold chain is broken. Seek advice from a pharmacist or the vaccine manufacturers in such an event.

Recommendations for vaccine storage are as shown below.[11]

Action	Rationale
A named person to be responsible for vaccines	To ensure the regulations are followed
Check and record min./max. temperatures daily	To ensure the correct temperature has been maintained throughout the 24 hours and as proof of regular monitoring

(Continued)

Action (continued)	Rationale (continued)
Defrost fridge regularly if not self-defrosting	For the most efficient and cost-efficient running
Store vaccines in a cold box or other fridge while defrosting	To maintain the cold chain
Make sure the fridge is wired in or has a dedicated socket, clearly marked	So it cannot be turned off accidentally
Make sure the fridge door closes properly	To maintain the correct temperature at all times
Do not load more than 50% of the fridge and allow room between batches on each shelf	Temperatures are maintained more easily if air can circulate freely
Do not stockpile vaccines and make sure that those delivered earliest are used before more recent ones	To ensure they are not kept too long or pass their expiry date
Do not store food or anything other than vaccines in the vaccine fridge	To reduce the need to open the fridge door unnecessarily and to comply with health and safety regulations
Ensure that a maintenance programme is in place for the vaccine fridge	To reduce the likelihood of breakdown and increase the efficiency and life of the fridge

Control of infection

Measures to prevent the spread of infection are needed in general practice. People who might be infectious should be tactfully taken to a waiting area away from other patients, and staff members who are ill ought to stay at home when necessary. Immunisation against influenza is offered to front line NHS staff and take-up should be encouraged. The practice should have a control of infection policy and appropriate training provided.

Hand washing

Sinks with elbow taps, soap dispensers and paper towels are needed in all the toilets and clinical areas to reduce hand-to-hand contamination. Bacteria have been shown to multiply on soap bars and reusable towels[12]. They are a possible source of cross-contamination and should not be used in clinical settings. Alcohol and chlorhexidine rub can be used on socially-clean hands if appropriate. Antiseptic handwash (e.g. Hibiscrub) should be used prior to invasive procedures[13].

Protective clothing

Disposable aprons should be worn for procedures likely to contaminate clothing. Gloves are needed when there is any risk of transmitting or contracting any infection. Sterile gloves must be used for invasive procedures such as minor surgery or inserting IUDs, and for dressing major wounds such as burns. Unsterile latex gloves are adequate for phlebotomy, minor dressings, and performing rectal or vaginal examinations. Powder free gloves are recommended to reduce the risk of latex allergy[14]. Non-latex gloves will be needed if a patient or staff member is sensitive to latex. Masks and eye protection should be available if there is any risk of blood being splashed into the mouth or eyes. Such risks are uncommon in general practice but if a risk is present then facilities for eye irrigation are also needed.

All the staff need to be familiar with the procedure for dealing with body fluids when accidents occur. Although HIV infection causes the most concern, the virus is less easily transmitted than hepatitis B. Much smaller amounts of hepatitis B virus are needed for infection and it is stable in organic matter outside the body for long periods.

Hepatitis B infection

The virus is spread by contact with infected body fluids through inoculation or contact with mucous membranes or broken skin. Any cuts or breaks in the skin should be covered with waterproof plaster. Clinical staff and phlebotomists need to be immunised against hepatitis B and have their immunity checked. A record should be kept of the immunisation dates and checks of antibody levels. There should also be a practice policy on needlestick injuries.

Human immunodeficiency virus (HIV) infection

Three factors must apply before HIV can be transmitted:

- Amount – there must be enough of the virus. HIV can be found in high concentrations in blood, semen and vaginal secretions of infected people. Sweat, tears, saliva, urine and faeces contain much less concentrated amounts.
- Condition – HIV deteriorates rapidly outside the body and is destroyed by heat, bleach and detergents. The enzymes in saliva and gastric acid also attack the virus.
- Route of infection – there must be a way into the bloodstream.

The most common means of spread are by unprotected sexual intercourse, sharing unclean equipment for IV drug use, or from mother to child. Infected blood inside a used needle could be injected during a needlestick injury. HIV has on rare occasions been contracted by individuals with severe eczema. The macrophages in the exudate of the eczematous lesions are thought to have ingested the virus in infected blood in contact with the skin.

Practice nurses have a role in educating people about HIV infection. That means separating the myths from the facts and having up-to-date knowledge. HIV/AIDS awareness days are regularly run locally by trusts and social service training departments. HIV/AIDS specialist nurses will provide guidance if asked.

Needlestick injuries

A strick adherence to the procedure for the use of sharps will prevent all but the most untoward accidents. If a needlestick injury occurs the following action should be taken immediately.

Action	Rationale
Encourage the puncture wound to bleed freely and wash under running water	To flush any organisms from the wound
Prevent squeezing or sucking of the sound	A vacuum effect may draw organisms inwards or hepatitis B virus could be ingested
Irrigate any mucous membranes exposed with plenty of water; wash eyes before and after removing contact lenses (if worn)	Micro-organisms can gain entry through aerosols of blood in contact with mucous membranes
Report the injury immediately to the employer	An accident report will be needed and tests may have to be performed
Ask the patient to wait (if known)	Blood bests may be requested (tests may be performed, with consent, for hepatitis B but counselling is needed before testing for HIV antibodies)
Blood may be taken from the person injured	As a baseline against later tests for hepatitis B and HIV
Immunisation against hepatitis B may be needed	(See Chapter 10)

Disinfection and sterilisation

Every practice should have a policy for the decontamination of equipment. The current guidelines are extensive but nevertheless, practices should be aware of them because they have a duty to comply. Central sterile supply (CSS) is the ideal way of ensuring a regular standard of sterile equipment but the service may be unavailable to some practices. The correct use of benchtop steam sterilisers is costly in both time and running costs. Single-use disposable items should be used whenever possible and these items must never be reprocessed[15]. The practice nurse is usually responsible for decontaminating non-disposable surgical and examination equipment. A thorough understanding of the principles is needed. Equipment may be treated according to the level of risk. For example:

- Low risk – aural specula, jet tip nozzles (used for irrigating non-infected ears)
- Moderate risk – vaginal specula, practice diaphragms, aural specula and irrigation nozzles (used for infected ears)
- High risk – minor surgery instruments and instruments for inserting IUDs.

Cleansing

All washable equipment must be thoroughly cleaned with hot water and detergent, and rinsed thoroughly. Household gloves and a disposal apron and eye protection should be worn, and splashing avoided. Blood or debris dried on the surface of an instrument will prevent adequate sterilisation. The use of ultrasonic baths with enzymatic solution is recommended to ensure the instruments are thoroughly clean[16]. Brushes used for cleaning equipment must be autoclaved, stored dry, and replaced regularly.

Sterilisation

Sterilisation destroys micro-organisms and spores and is the only safe method of decontamination for high-risk instruments. If a CSSD service is not available, autoclaving is the most effective method of sterilisation in general practice[17].

Autoclaves This process uses steam under pressure to sterilise instruments and other equipment. Autoclaves can be obtained in different sizes, but they are required to meet the standards laid down in the Medical Devices Regulations[18-19]. Sterilisation may be achieved with a high temperature for a short period or with longer cycles at lower temperatures. In order to be effective the appropriate temperature must be maintained for the correct length of time. The times taken to reach a temperature and to cool down afterwards are immaterial.

Sterilisation times at different temperatures are shown in Table 4.1.

The reservoir should be filled with sterile water for irrigation, which should be changed daily. In reality, many practices still use distilled water but nurses

Table 4.1 Sterilisation times at different temperatures.

Temperature	Holding time
134–137°C	3 minutes
126–129°C	10 minutes
121–124°C	15 minutes

should be aware of the recommendations. These also include four-monthly servicing, with emergency repairs as necessary and additional daily and weekly checks by the user[20]. Details of the temperature and holding times must be logged; ideally from a print-out of the sterilisation data, which all newer autoclaves have. The steam must be able to reach all the surfaces of an object. The blades of instruments must be open, and overloading of the trays avoided. Gallipots and receivers should be placed on their side. Instruments can be sterilised in pouches only in vacuum autoclaves. Special racks are needed to keep the pouches separate and in a vertical position. If practice diaphragms are to be reused, they may be autoclaved but the drying cycle must be omitted. Chaetle forceps should be kept in a clean, dry holder next to the autoclave and be used only for removing sterilised objects. The forceps should be autoclaved at least once daily and prior to setting minor surgery and IUD trolleys.

A practice policy is needed to ensure contaminated equipment is never put into the autoclave until ready to start the sterilisation process. That way, unsterile equipment cannot be taken out of the autoclave and reused by mistake.

Disinfection

Chemical disinfectants and boiling water can destroy bacteria and other microorganisms but do not destroy spores.

Chemical disinfection   Chemicals may be used for low and medium risk items like thermometers and items which cannot be autoclaved. Glutaraldehyde, used in hospital to disinfect endoscopes, should not be used in general practice. Glutaraldehyde produces toxic fumes which can cause occupational asthma and dermatitis, so special procedures are needed to comply with the COSHH regulations[21]. Alcohol and chlorine releasing products are most commonly used in general practice. Industrial alcohol can be used to disinfect clean, heat-sensitive items. Twenty minutes immersion time is needed. Sodium hypochlorite, as household bleach or Milton can be used in dilution for 30 minutes to disinfect plastics and glass. Sodium dichloroisocyanurate (NaDCC) tablets, e.g. Haz Tabs or Presept, can be dissolved in water to give a more reliable dilution of chlorine. The dilutions needed depend on the brand. The instructions on the label should be followed. Plastic injection trays, aural specula, ear irrigation nozzles, and bowls used to wash feet, are suitable for this treatment. Each day before use, the electric ear irrigator should be cleaned with NaDCC solution as follows:

- Fill the machine's tank with the solution
- Run the machine to pump the solution through the tubing, turn off and leave to stand for ten minutes
- Empty the tank, refill with tap water and pump it through the tubing to rinse it

- Disinfect the machine at the end of the day, rinse with sterile water and pump it through the tubing; dry the machine well.
(Advice from the Primary Ear Care Centre)

NaDCC granules (Presept) can be used to disinfect blood and other body fluids. All the staff should be aware of the procedure if a spillage occurs, as outlined below.

Action	Rationale
Wear household rubber gloves	To avoid hand contact
Cover the spillage with chlorine granules or a 1% hypochlorite solution; leave for ten minutes	To inactivate any organisms
Remove any broken glass with forceps	To avoid accidental cuts
Cover the spillage with paper towels or use scoop in the special spillage kit, if available, to transfer the spillage to a yellow bag	For incineration as clinical waste
Use hot water and strong detergent for surfaces, such as carpets	Where bleach would cause damage to the fabric

The disposal of clinical waste

The Environment Protection Act (1990) requires everybody who produces clinical waste to ensure that:

- The waste is stored correctly until collected
- A written description of the waste is supplied
- The waste is transferred by a registered carrier.

Blades, needles and syringes must be deposited in sharps containers which meet the British Standard BS 7320:1990. The containers should be assembled correctly and placed appropriately, so that sharps can be safely disposed of close to their point of use. The containers must be kept out of reach of children because sadly, accidents have been known to occur whereby children sustained needlestick injuries through reaching into used sharps bins.

Dressings and other soft waste contaminated with blood or body fluids must go into yellow bags contained in foot operated pedal bins. Used bags must be tied securely with a special plastic fastener. The sharps bins and yellow bags must be stored in a locked room, cupboard or a yellow wheelie bin, inaccessible to the public. The waste must be able to be traced back to the person responsible and so must carry a label with the practice address and date of disposal. Unwanted medicines must also be disposed of safely to comply with the terms of the Environment Protection Act. On one occasion a GP was prosecuted and found to be negligent after the drugs given to a pharmacist for disposal were found dumped[21]. The practice must have a contract for a regular collection of the clinical waste. On no account must it be put into the ordinary rubbish bins.

Supplies and equipment

The amount of clinical equipment needed varies from practice to practice (see Appendix 1). The practice nurse is responsible for overseeing the proper upkeep and for knowing the correct way to use the equipment in his/her care. Instruction booklets and guarantees should be kept on file. Any faulty equipment must be withdrawn from use, labelled and reported to the practice manager or GP. Maintenance contracts are needed for essential or potentially dangerous items such as autoclaves.

Emergency equipment

Every practice must have a basic supply of emergency drugs and equipment kept easily accessible. The exact items to be kept should be agreed by the clinicians. The practice nurse is usually responsible for ensuring that emergency supplies are checked and maintained. Epinephrine (adrenaline) has a relatively short shelf-life and will need to be replaced regularly. All items must be purchased initially but reimbursement can be claimed for any personally administered drugs (see Appendix 2, Emergency equipment).

Ordering supplies and equipment

Practice policy will determine who has the responsibility for ordering supplies. Whether nurses place orders directly or via the practice manager, everyone has a responsibility for seeking value for money. Discounts may be available for bulk orders but it can be a false economy if the items do not have a long enough shelf-life. Some items may appear cheaper by mail order but small orders can attract expensive delivery charges. Some examples of sources of supply are shown in Table 4.2. Copies of requisitions and receipts need to be kept for reference and accounting purposes.

Training in emergency procedures

Resuscitation

As many practice staff as possible should be able to undertake basic life-support measures in emergencies. People tend to go to the surgery in times of

Table 4.2   Sources of supply.

Source	Product examples
Direct purchase from manufacturer	Travel vaccines
Purchase from wholesaler or medical mail order firm	Examination and diagnostic equipment, injections, gloves, paper goods, dressings, IUDs, diaphragms, drugs
Purchase on account from local pharmacy	Small quantity items needed quickly
On prescription from local pharmacy	Dressings and drugs for named patients
Requisition from the health authority/primary care agency	Syringes, needles, NHS stationery
Requisition from district hospital	Pathology forms and sample bottles
Requisition from Farillon	Childhood and routine vaccines
Local health promotion department	Leaflets, posters, videos etc. for health promotion and patient information
Contract with clinical waste service	Yellow bags and sharps bins

trouble but there may not always be a doctor or other nurse in the building. Resuscitation training can usually be arranged through the local trust's resuscitation training officer. Regular updating is also needed (see Chapter 7, Emergency Situations).

Fire precautions

Every practice should have a procedure for dealing with a fire and an adequate supply of appropriate fire extinguishers, together with a map or plan of their location. Extinguishers must be serviced at least once annually and staff trained in their use at a full fire practice.

Suggestions for reflection on practice

- Review all the storage and disposal facilities in the nurses' rooms. Do they meet all the legal requirements and comply with local guidelines?
- Review:
  - The facilities for patient care in the nurses' rooms. Are they satisfactory?
  - The procedures for decontaminating and sterilising equipment in your practice. Prepare a report, including appropriate references, if any changes are needed.

- Liaise with the practice manager to organise an emergency procedure practice. Assess the results:
  - Did everyone know what to do?
  - Was all the emergency equipment available and in working order?
  - Could anything have been done better?

Further reading

May, D. and Brewer, S. (2001) Sharps injury: prevention and management. *Nursing Standard*, **15** (32), 45–52.

Memel, D. and Francis, K. (2001) Disability. *Practice Nurse*, **21** (8), 21–3.

Royal College of Nursing factsheet (2000) *Universal Precautions for the Control of Infection*. Royal College of Nursing, London.

Royal College of Nursing and NHS Executive (1998) *Safer Working in the Community: a guide for NHS managers and staff on reducing the risk from violence and aggression*. RCN, London.

References

1. Parliament (1995) *Disability Discrimination Act, 1995*, Section 21. HMSO, London.
2. NHS Health Development Agency (2001) *New Primary Care Premises*. Health Development Agency, London.
3. Moore, R. & Moore, S. (1995) *Health and Safety at Work. Guidance for General Practitioners*. Royal College of General Practitioners, London.
4. Watchdog Healthcheck Report – Toys (26/6/00) BBC Online. *www.bbc.co.ik/watchdog/reports/health/hctoys* (accessed 8/9/01).
5. Parliament (1974) *Health and Safety at Work ETC (HSW) Act, 1974*. HMSO, London.
6. Statutory Instrument (1992) No. 273. *Manual Handling Operations Regulations 1992*. HMSO, London.
7. Health and Safety Executive *Control of Substances Hazardous to Health Regulations* (1988), made under the *Health and Safety at Work Act 1974*. HMSO, London.
8. British Hypertension Society Information Service. *Blood Pressure Monitors*, *www.hyp.ac.uk/bhsinfo/bpmindex* (accessed 8/9/01).
9. Destruction of controlled drugs in *BMA briefing – Conviction of Harold Shipman*. British Medical Association Online, *www.bma.org.uk/public/pubother.nsf/webdocssvw/shipmanbriefing* (accessed 7/9/01).
10. News item (1992) Doctor faces charge after child drank acid. *Daily Telegraph*, 19 September 1996.
11. Grassby, P. (1992) *Safe Storage of Vaccines: Problems and solutions*. St Mary's Hospital, Penarth, S. Glamorgan.
12. Mendes, M. & Lynch, D. (1976) A bacteriological survey of washrooms and toilets. *Journal of Hygiene*, **76**, 183–90.
13. Gould, D. (2000) Hand decontamination. *Nursing Standard*, **15** (6), 45–9.

14. Health Service Circular HSC 1999/186 (1999). *Latex medical gloves and powdered latex medical gloves*. NHS Executive, Leeds.
15. Royal College of Nursing (Reprinted 2001) *Good Practice in Infection Control – guidance for nurses working in general practice*. Royal College of Nursing, London.
16. Amendment to the *Consumer Protection Act 1987* by the Medical Devices Regulations (SI 1994 No 3017).
17. Amendment is the *Consumer Protection Act 1987* by the Medical Devices Regulations (SI 1994 No 3017).
18. Pressure Systems and Transportable Gas Containers Regulations 1989 (SI 1989/2169).
19. Medical Devices Agency (2000) *Guidance on the Purchase, Operation and Maintenance of Benchtop Steam Sterilizers*. MDA DB 2000 (05).
20. Health and Safety Executive (1998) *Chemical Hazard Alert Notice – Glutaraldehyde*. HSE, Sheffield.
21. Disposal of unwanted medicines (1993) *Journal of the Medical Defence Union*, **9** (4), 79.

Useful addresses and web sites

Medical Devices Agency
20 Hannibal House, Elephant and Castle, London SE1 6TQ
Telephone 020 7972 8000
Web site: *www.medical-devices.gov.uk*

NHS Plus – Occupational Health Service for smaller employers
Web site: *nhsplus@doh.gsi.gov.uk*

Chapter 5
Nursing Treatments and Procedures

The importance to the patients of hands-on nursing care should never be overlooked as the role of nurses changes and expands. Patients are entitled to care that is based on the best available evidence of effectiveness. Thoughtful preparation and skilled performance can minimise the discomfort caused by many nursing procedures and even apparently routine tasks provide opportunities for health promotion and active listening to patients' concerns.

Injections

A variety of injections are given in general practice (specific injections are dealt with in the relevant chapters). Injections are usually prescribed by a doctor, either in the patient's records or on a prescription form. Immunisations may be given under a patient group direction. Injection techniques are taught in pre-registration training and will not be described here.

A badge or certificate of bravery will console many children after an injection. Feeding seems to be the best pacifier for young babies, while a bright, musical toy will usually distract older infants. Anaesthetic cream is available on prescription and can be applied to the injection site, with an occlusive dressing, one hour before injection for very nervous children, or those who require a large number of injections.

Records must be kept of the product name, dose, route of administration, manufacturer, batch number and expiry date. This applies to any medicine – not just injections. A nurse or doctor could be legally responsible for any harm to a patient, if unable to prove the source of the product used[1]. The site of injection should also be recorded, especially when more than one injection is given; in case of an adverse reaction to any product. The injection data may also be needed for immunisation targets or for a recall system. The nurse must observe the patient until satisfied that there are no immediate ill effects from the injection. It is not possible to specify an exact time. Some practice policies state a minimum time of 20 minutes. Patients need information about possible side effects and the action to take if they occur. The summary of product characteristics list all the possible adverse reactions. There is usually a portion to be given to the patient and a part for the professional who is administering the product. Patients receiving regular injections should know when to make the next appointment. A recall system may be needed for immunisations or depot medication.

Wound care

Practice nurses are likely to encounter patients with a variety of wounds. The range of dressings can be bewildering and sales representatives produce convincing arguments for favouring their own products. A sound understanding of the principles of wound healing is necessary when selecting a dressing. A local trust wound care specialist will provide education and advice if needed. Some areas have wound product formularies which can make the selection process easier.

Wound healing

There are three distinct phases of healing, although some overlap occurs between them:

- *Inflammation* in response to the initial injury. A fibrin clot forms, to prevent further blood loss. Blood vessels in the vicinity of the wound become more permeable and leukocytes are attracted to the area to remove bacteria and debris by phagocytosis. (The normal inflammatory response, which causes slight redness around a wound, should not be mistaken for infection.)

- *Proliferation* of cells and collagen. Fibroblasts produce collagen fibres, and buds of endothelial cells and capillaries grow into the wound space to form the delicate granulation tissue. Occasionally over-granulation can occur above the level of the surrounding skin. This can usually be arrested by a pressure dressing or application of a steroid cream.

- *Maturation* as the wound heals. Epithelial cells migrate across the wound until it is covered. Collagen is broken down and remoulded over subsequent months to form a firmer scar. Keloid forms when there is an overproduction of collagen. Patients with dark skin are more prone to developing keloid scars[2].

Wounds are often classified according to their appearance or stage of healing:

- *Necrotic wounds* – when devitalised tissue forms a dry, hard, black eschar, or a soft, grey slough. Surgical or chemical debridement is necessary.

- *Infected wounds* – when bacteria overcome the body's natural defences. There may be a purulent discharge and/or cellulitis present. Systemic antibiotics may be needed. All wounds become colonised by bacteria, but are not necessarily infected[3].

- *Clean wounds* – are those without slough or infection. They may be superficial or deep. The skin margins of incisions may be drawn together to reduce the gap to be bridged. Wider wounds heal by granulation.

Necrotic or infected tissue delays healing and must be treated. Sterile larvae (maggots) have been used to good effect in desloughing wounds. The larvae and information about their application can be obtained from the Biosurgical Research Unit. Wounds usually heal more quickly in the warm, moist environment created by an occlusive dressing because the epithelial cells can migrate across the wound rather than growing downwards under a scab[4]. However, the risk of infection in patients with diabetes could be so devastating that some diabetologists are opposed to occlusive dressings for neuropathic and ischaemic ulcers in their patients.

Dressings

The dressing range available on prescription includes:

- *Sterile dressing packs* which open to provide a sterile field and contain a handtowel/paper drape, four cotton wool balls, four gauze swabs and a dressing pad. The packs are expensive and may not be needed for minor dressings. (Cotton wool is not recommended in wound cleansing because fibres can be left in the wound and impair healing.) Packs of five sterile gauze swabs, or 100 unsterile swabs are also available on prescription and may be more cost effective than dressing packs.

- *Normal saline* is used as single-use 25 ml units for irrigating wounds. Tap water is more economical and has been shown to be safe for wound cleansing[5]. Antiseptics can damage fragile granulation tissue and are generally contraindicated.

- *Enzyme preparations* can be used to debride necrotic tissue. The preparation is expensive, but it can last a little longer if mixed with KY jelly and stored in the refrigerator.

- *Hydrocolloid dressings* – waterproof adhesive wafers which combine with exudate from a wound to form a gel; useful for desloughing wounds and promoting granulation. Hydrocolloid paste can be used in deep wounds and sinuses. They may cause over-granulation if they are used for too long. The liquid which forms under the wafer can be mistaken for pus. The offensive odour of the liquid and leakage can distress patients. Skin maceration can occur if there is excessive exudate.

- *Hydrogels* – a soft gel packaged in dispenser units, which can be applied directly to a wound and covered with a film or secondary dressing. The gel helps to rehydrate wounds and create the optimum conditions for healing. It has a range of uses similar to hydrocolloids.

- *Calcium alginate dressings* are made of an extract of seaweed spun and woven into soft mats and are useful as a haemostat and for absorbing exudate. This can be used under occlusive films or other secondary dressings. They can be removed from wounds by saline irrigation. The dressings sometimes stick fast but soaking with saline will work, with patience. Cavity-packing material is also produced.

- *Polyurethane foam* absorbs exudate through the non-adherent contact layer into the foam backing. It can be used under compression bandages, and as a light, comfortable dressing for arterial ulcers. The foam can be cut easily and makes a good dressing after toenail surgery. It is useful for controlling over-granulation.

- *Vapour-permeable film dressings* can be used to secure a dressing or to provide a warm, moist environment for clean, superficial wounds. It is also useful for keeping enzymatic preparations moist. Some patients are allergic to the adhesive. Skin can be damaged if the film is pulled away. It should be lifted and stretched off the skin.

- *Non-adherent dressings* are thin wound contact dressings designed not to stick to wounds. They can be used for venous ulcers under compression bandages and are also useful for minor burns with silver sulphadiazine cream. Secondary dressings are needed. Dressings made of this material and impregnated with povidone iodine are available.

Impregnated gauzes have limited uses. Paraffin gauze might be used occasionally on skin graft sites or for minor burns. Allergic reactions to impregnated gauzes can occur.

Strapping and bandages

These may be applied to secure a dressing, to give support or provide compression to an underlying structure.

Adhesive tape can be used to secure dressings, or for neighbour-strapping injured fingers and toes. Many people are allergic to zinc oxide adhesive and it can be difficult to remove.

Microporous tape is light, hypoallergenic and easy to remove. Some patients can still become allergic to the adhesive. The tape is used to secure dressings, but it does not stretch as the body moves. Strips of sterile reinforced microporous tape (Steri-strips) can be used to close minor incisions and cuts. Reimbursement of prescriptions can be claimed for these as personally administered items.

Paper-backed tape (Hypafix, Mepore) is not available on prescription, but is a light, stretchable fixative, which if used sensibly, is very useful and not too expensive to buy. A range of sizes of all-in-one dressings, made of this of tape with non-adhesive pads, (Mepore, Primapore), can be prescribed.

Conforming bandages are light, loosely woven bandages for securing dressings. The edges can cut into oedematous tissue if applied too tightly, and those with elastic fibres can cause oedema above and below the bandage if it is over-extended.

Tubular gauze comes in a range of sizes, and can hold dressings in place, or be used under bandages to protect sensitive skin. The small sizes are useful for dressing fingers and toes. Applicators are available in a range of sizes.

Tubular elastic bandages in sizes B to G, provide support for soft tissue injuries. It is designed to be used in a double layer. Special measuring tapes can be obtained from the manufacturers for assessing the size needed.

Crepe bandages can be used to secure dressings or to provide support for soft tissue injuries.

Paste bandages can be used in conjunction with compression bandages to treat venous ulcers. Severe allergies to some of the constituents can develop. A skin test is recommended before applying a paste bandage. Paste bandages may also be used for treating severe eczema[6].

Elastic crepe bandages provide support but quickly lose their elasticity. Tuition and practice is needed to get the correct amount of extension when applying them.

Four layer bandages are now available on prescription (see venous ulcers below).

Compression hosiery can be prescribed for individual patients. There are three classes of compression:

- Class I gives the least compression
- Class II gives the moderate compression needed for most patients in general practice
- Class III is for very firm compression.

The stockings can have closed or open toes and be knee or thigh length. Black support hose are available for men, and made to measure hose can be prescribed for patients with unusual measurements.

General assessment of the patient

Wound care entails much more than applying dressings. A full assessment is needed. The factors to consider include:

- *Age*   Elderly patients have slower rates of growth and repair, less collagen and elasticity in the skin, and may have impaired circulation. The immune system can also be less effective. Care is needed to avoid damaging fragile skin with adhesives or tight bandages.

- *Mobility*   Patients who are not very mobile are more likely to develop oedema or to fall. Referrals for physiotherapy or occupational therapy may be needed to help to improve mobility. Housebound patients may need to be referred to the district nurse for treatment.

- *Nutritional state*   Obesity can contribute to reduced mobility and make bandaging difficult. Malnourished or cachexic patients can lack the vitamins and minerals needed for wound healing. Patients may need information about healthy eating. Those who are unable to eat a healthy diet may require food supplements or need to see a dietitian. Protein intake can be checked by liver function tests (albumin levels).

- *Medical conditions*   The general medical condition can influence the progress of any wound. Anaemia, diabetes, rheumatoid arthritis, immunosuppression, and cardiopulmonary disease can all contribute to the development or continuation of tissue damage. A doctor should be consulted when necessary.

- *Psychological state*   The patient's motivation should be assessed. Patients may lack the energy or inclination to care for themselves properly, or they may have self-inflicted injuries. Counselling and/or antidepressant therapy may be needed.

- *Social situation*   Lonely patients have sometimes been suspected of exacerbating their wounds to maintain contact with the nurse. Referrals may be made to social services or voluntary agencies to arrange other contacts.

- *Smoking*   Smoking reduces the amount of oxygen available to the tissues, and increases the damage to small blood vessels[7].

- *Alcohol intake*   A high alcohol intake can adversely affect the nutritional state and cause damage to the liver and kidneys.

- *Pain*   Pain may limit mobility or affect sleep. Analgesics might be needed, and the choice of dressing can be influenced if the wound is very painful.

The assessment and treatment of the wound

The wound assessment should include: the type, size, stage of healing, amount of exudate, and any complicating factors. The possibility of malignancy should be borne in mind in any wound which fails to heal or looks suspicious. Measurements of the wound provide an objective scale against which to judge progress. Tracing over a double plastic film is a quick, easy method which allows the top layer to be kept free from contamination by the wound. Photographs also provide a good reference. A ruler should be included in the picture to show the scale.

Choice of dressing

Considerations when choosing a dressing include:

- Practical issues – getting shoes on, bathing, frequency of dressing changes, patient concordance
- Aesthetic factors – how the dressings looks, feels, smells
- Cost – an important issue but should not deter the use of the most suitable product.

Wound care is most effective if the patient is involved in planning the treatment and lifestyle changes necessary to promote healing. Advice may be sought from a wound care adviser if a wound poses particular difficulties. The possibility of malignancy should always be considered if a wound fails to heal or is recurrent.

Leg ulcers

Leg ulcers, often painful and debilitating to patients, use vast resources in manpower and dressings annually. The correct diagnosis of the ulcer type is essential before treatment is started.

Arterial ulcers

Arterial ulcers result from ischaemia due to arterial occlusion; often caused by atherosclerosis. Minor trauma may cause an ulcer to develop and the tissue breaks down as a result of impaired supply of oxygen and nutrients. Smoking exacerbates the problem.

Recognition   This will include:

- Position of the ulcer – often below the ankle
- Appearance – often well-demarcated, deep, with a pale base, necrosis and absence of healthy granulation tissue; the skin around the ulcer may be shiny and dry, and the toenails thickened
- Pain – particularly at night, often severe
- Foot pulses – may be absent or diminished (experience is needed to locate foot pulses, *not an accurate indicator*). Assessment of arterial bloodflow by Doppler ultrasound is more objective, and early referral for arteriography should be made, if appropriate.

Aims of treatment   These will include:

- To reduce pain
- To assist healing
- To prevent further tissue damage.

Treatment	Rationale
Ensure that the patient has adequate analgesia and knows when to take it	Ischaemic ulcers can be very painful
Identify any contributing medical conditions	Diabetes, rheumatoid arthritis, anaemia and malignancy may contribute to ischaemic ulcers
Arrange for systemic antibiotics if needed	Infection may delay healing
Apply suitable light dressings	For lightness, comfort and ease of removal and to encourage healing
Avoid compression bandages	To avoid compromising the circulation further
Encourage smoking cessation	To avoid further vascular damage and to improve the oxygen supply to the tissues

Surgery may be indicated to try and improve the blood-flow for patients with ischaemic. In extreme cases amputation can become necessary.

Venous ulcers

Venous ulcers result from inadequacy of the venous drainage of the legs. Incompetent valves in the perforator veins allow a back-flow and increased venous pressure in the superficial veins.

Recognition   This will include noting the following:

- Skin condition – in varicose eczema, brown discolouration is caused by the breakdown of red blood cells in the tissues
- Ulcer position – commonest in the gaiter area, the pre-tibial and antero-medial supra-malleolar areas
- Appearance – superficial with uneven edges and some granulation tissue
- Oedema due to venous insufficiency; often exacerbated by reduced mobility
- Pain: ulcers may be very painful, although patients can sometimes be pain-free.

Doppler assessment plays an essential part in the diagnosis of venous ulcers.

Aims of treatment   These will include:

- To improve the venous return and reduce stagnation in the tissues of the affected leg
- To provide clear information and encouragement to enable the patient to participate in the treatment and to maintain his/her legs in their optimum condition after healing has occurred.

Treatment	Rationale
Wash the leg ulcer with warm water	To remove debris without damaging the wound surface or cooling the wound
Apply a flat, non-irritant, non-adherent dressing or a hydrocolloid wafer	To prevent indentation of the surrounding skin and allow removal of the dressing without damage to healing tissues
Pad smoothly with absorbent material	To absorb exudate and protect the bony prominences
Apply graduated compression bandages (needs to be sustained at 40 mmHg at the ankle[8])	To reverse venous hypertension without compromising the arterial circulation
Advise elevation of the foot above the level of the hip when resting	To reduce oedema by using gravity
Teach suitable ankle exercises (dorsi flexing and plantar flexing the feet, and circular movements of the ankles)	To aid the venous return by the action of the calf muscle pump and aid mobility
Teach the need to prevent a recurrence by good skin care, the use of compression hosiery and early treatment of injury	Patients who understand their condition can take responsibility for looking after their legs and for getting help when needed

Compression bandaging cannot be learned from a book. Expert tuition and practice in four-layer bandaging is needed. Moreover, no patient should have compression bandages applied without having had a Doppler assessment.

Mixed ulcers

Some patients have mixed ulcers caused by both arterial and venous insufficiency. Compression must be avoided where there is any risk to the arterial blood flow.

Eye treatments

Patients may ask to see the practice nurse with various eye conditions. Nurses are advised to err on the side of caution and refer to the GP when in any doubt about dealing with eye conditions.

The principles of eye care are:

Action	Rationale
Avoid using antiseptic spray on the hands	It can cause irritation to the patient's eyes
Ensure there is a good light source	To be able to assess the eye properly and avoid injury during any eye treatment
Avoid shining the light directly into the eye	The patient may have photophobia
Tell the patient what action is proposed	To avoid sudden movements which could injure the eye and to obtain informed consent
Inspect the eye for signs of infection, allergy foreign body or injury	To identify the problem and ensure the correct treatment is given
Enquire about the patient's vision; check visual acuity if necessary (see Chapter 6)	In case of any abnormality which needs investigation

(See Chapter 7 under eye problems for foreign bodies in the eye, conjunctivitis, corneal abrasions and painful eyes).

Ear care

Ear irrigation, still called syringing by many people, is usually carried out by practice nurses for the removal of excessive earwax. Softening drops should be recommended for use at least three days beforehand. Olive oil is considered to be preferable to proprietary drops or sodium bicarbonate. Patients with impacted wax may need to use the drops for longer. Occasionally patients may require ear irrigation to remove debris or a foreign body from the auditory canal. The procedure should not be attempted for any hygroscopic foreign body, such as a pea, which is likely to swell in contact with water.

Any practice nurse who undertakes ear irrigation must have had adequate training and supervision to ensure that patients are not harmed. The Primary Ear Care Centre in Rotherham runs a course in ear care accredited by Sheffield University. Ear care trainers run satellite courses and study days around the country. The protocol should specify the circumstances under which patients may self-refer for treatment and the contraindications to irrigation. Such contraindications include:

- A recent history of otalgia or otitis media
- A recent history of discharging ears or current tympanic membrane perforation
- If there were untoward experiences following ear syringing in the past
- If the patient has grommets in situ
- If the patient has a cleft palate, even if repaired

- *Never* irrigate a mastoid cavity
- If a patient has deafness in one ear, damage caused by irrigation of the hearing ear could be devastating: it is recommended that irrigation is not undertaken for such patients[10].

Metal ear syringes should not be used at all. Electric pulsed water units are safer and less likely to cause damage to the ear. Problems caused by ear syringing were reported by the Medical Defence Union as being the second highest reason, over a five-year period, for claims for negligence involving procedures performed by doctors and nurses[11].

As with any nursing procedure, a full history and examination are needed before starting the treatment. Both ears should be examined with the auriscope and the necessity for irrigation decided. It is not uncommon for patients with dysfunction of the middle ear to present for ear syringing because their ears feel 'blocked'. The skin of the auditory canal will sometimes be inflamed or itchy; particularly in patients who have skin conditions such as eczema or psoriasis. Irritation or allergic reactions can also result from the use of proprietary cerumolytic drops.

Equipment needed

The following equipment will be required:

- head light or head mirror and lamp
- plastic cape and towel
- auriscope
- electric pulsed water unit with clean jet nozzle
- specially shaped receiver (Noots tank)
- Jobson Horne probe
- cotton wool
- tissues
- receivers for used tissues, cotton wool and instruments.

Procedure

The patient and nurse should both be seated and the entire procedure should be carried out under direct vision, using a head light or head mirror and lamp.

(1) Check whether the patient has had his/her ears syringed previously and identify any contraindications to the procedure.
(2) Explain the procedure to the patient, in order to obtain informed consent, and to ensure that the patient will not be unduly anxious and will remain still during the procedure.
(3) Ask the patient to sit in the examination chair with their head tilted to allow visualisation of the auditory meatus. (A child could sit on an adult's lap with the child's head held steady.)

(4) Inspect the ear to be syringed, with the auriscope. The other ear should also be inspected for comparison.

(5) Place the protective cape and towel in position and ask the patient to hold the receiver under the ear.

(6) Fill the reservoir of the pulsed water unit with water at body temperature (38°C). Deviations in temperature can cause dizziness by causing convection currents in the semicircular canals.

(7) Put on the head light or head mirror, turn on the light and adjust as necessary.

(8) Ensure that the jet tip is firmly attached to the holder, set the pressure to the appropriate setting, aim the jet tip into the receiver and switch on the machine.

(9) Run any cold water or air out of the tubing to ensure that any static water is discarded and only water at the correct temperature is used. This will also allow time for the patient to become accustomed to the sound of the machine.

(10) Twist the jet tip so that the water can be aimed in the right direction.

(11) Hold the pinna of the ear to be syringed with the non-dominant hand and pull gently upwards and backwards in an adult, or directly backwards if a child.

(12) Place the tip of the nozzle into the entrance of the external auditory meatus. Warn the patient that the procedure is about to start and to report any pain or dizziness, so that the procedure can be stopped immediately. Irrigation may cause discomfort but should *never* cause pain.

(13) Make sure that the entrance to the meatus is illuminated. Switch on the machine and direct the stream of water along the roof of the meatus towards the posterior wall, e.g. at the five minutes to the hour clock position for the right ear, and five minutes past the hour for the left ear. Turn the switch to increase the water pressure if necessary.

(14) Inspect the ear with the auriscope periodically and inspect the water running into the receiver.

(15) Dry mop excess water from the meatus under direct vision, using best quality cotton wool and the Jobson Horne probe. Stagnation of water and any abrasion of the skin during the procedure predisposes to otitis externa and possible *Pseudomonas* infection.

(16) Examine the meatus and tympanic membrane, and treat as required or refer to the GP if necessary.

(17) Record all findings and treatments in the patients clinical record.

(18) All the equipment used must be cleaned and disinfected (see Chapter 4).

Probably the most important part of the consultation is educating the patient about everyday ear care. The ears should be kept as dry as possible to allow the wax to migrate normally to the entrance of the auditory meatus. Attempting to clean the ears with cotton buds etc. should be avoided because this can cause the wax to become impacted and carries the risk of damage to the tympanic membrane as well.

Assisting with minor surgery

The advantages to patients of the growth of minor surgery in general practice include reduced waiting times for treatment and a more personal service in a familiar environment. Many doctors and nurses enjoy the chance to extend their professional skills. Although some nurses have been taught to perform some minor surgical procedures, it is still more usual for practice nurses to assist a GP with minor surgery. The standards of care required for performing minor surgery in general practice must include: the control of infection, the comfort and safety of the patient and the ability to deal with emergency situations.

The practice nurse's role

Preparation of the environment

The nurse has a responsibility for overseeing the high standard of cleanliness in the room used for minor surgery. The couch and lamp should be positioned to allow free access to the operation site. A comfortable room temperature is needed. Curtains or blinds should be adjusted to give privacy to patients.

Preparation of the equipment

Trolleys should be cleaned with soap and water and dried with paper towels. If CSSD packs are not available, the instruments must be sterilised and laid between sterile paper sheets; dressing packs are commonly used. Trolleys must not be laid up until ready to use because of the risk of contamination by micro-organisms. Some surgeries already use disposable scalpels and in the future it may become the norm for more disposable instruments to be used. Cost generally precludes this at the moment but fears about the spread of variant Creutzfeldt-Jakob disease may make this inevitable[12].

Preparation of the patient

Most people will experience some apprehension. Practice nurses can help by ensuring patients receive a clear explanation of what to expect and by encouraging the use of simple relaxation techniques. Patients commonly request to have moles and other skin lesions removed but are then surprised to learn that they will have a scar. The person performing the minor surgery is responsible for obtaining consent but the nurse can reinforce the information given. Each patient should be asked to remove clothing as necessary, to make sure the operation site is accessible. Clothing not removed should be protected from any possible blood trickles; even small lesions can be surprisingly vascular. If the operation site is on the scalp some hair may need to be trimmed but it may be possible just to tape hair out of the way. Eyebrows should not be shaved because they may not regrow.

During the operation

The nurse assisting should comfort and observe the patient during the minor operation and assist as needed, for example, by checking the local anaesthetic, opening sterile packs, receiving specimens for histology and assisting with suturing. The nurse will usually dress the wound and select the appropriate fixative.

After the operation

The patient may need time to recover before leaving the surgery. The nurse should ensure that the patient is able to get home safely and understands how to care for the wound, and when to return. Written advice sheets can be useful because verbal instructions are easily forgotten. The stress experienced by patients, undergoing what can seem to be trivial procedures, should never be underestimated.

Clearing up often falls to the nurse. Although the safe disposal of sharps is the responsibility of the person who used them, extreme caution is needed in case any have been overlooked. Items left on the bottom of trolleys can be hazardous to children, so trolleys must be cleared completely. Specimens for histology must be labelled and dispatched, with the appropriate form, to the laboratory.

Basic minor operation trolley

Each doctor may have favourite instruments but a basic set usually comprises:

- scalpel handle and blade or disposable scalpel
- two pairs of toothed dissecting forceps
- two pairs of non-toothed dissecting forceps
- curette
- artery forceps
- needle holder
- scissors
- sterile gallipot.

Also needed are: disposable apron, chlorhexidine hand scrub, sterile surgeons' gloves, local anaesthetic, syringes and needles, povidone iodine skin prep solution, specimen container and formaldehyde solution, suture materials, dressings and fixative. A silver nitrate stick or cautery may also be required.

The clinician's preferences will determine the equipment for specific procedures but some of the extra instruments and equipment include the following for each procedure.

Removal of sebaceous cysts

Curved scissors and mosquito forceps are used to dissect out a cyst and keep the capsule intact.

Incision of abscesses

- Equipment required includes ethylchloride spray (local anaesthetic) and a wound swab for microbiology.
- Instruments needed are sinus forceps or a probe.
- The dressing used will be alginate strip for light packing.
- Note: although it is good practice to ensure all patients undergoing minor surgery have had a routine urinalysis, boils, abscesses or carbuncles should raise particular suspicions about diabetes mellitus. A blood glucose test might be needed.

Ingrowing toenails

Wedge resection or removal of an ingrowing toenail may be necessary if conservative treatment is unsuccessful. Advice and information on footcare may help to prevent a recurrence.

Equipment required:

- Plain lignocaine 1% or 2% – as local anaesthetic for a ring block (adrenaline could cause gangrene of a digit through vasoconstriction)
- A tourniquet to reduce bleeding – can be made from a sterilised out-of-date unused catheter
- Instruments – sturdy, pointed scissors and a nail elevator
- Dressings need to be easily removable without causing pain, e.g. polyurethane foam, calcium alginate, or hydrocolloid.

Skin tags

Some papillomas may be removed surgically. Small skin tags can be tied tightly with suture silk, which usually causes them to necrose and drop off after a few days.

Warts and verrucae

Warts and verrucae are caused by the human papilloma virus, which accelerates the growth of the infected skin cells and distorts them. Most people eventually acquire an immunity to the virus but this can take months or years to develop. The correct diagnosis is essential before commencing treatment in the surgery. If proprietary treatments containing salicylic acid are unsuccessful, cryotherapy using liquid nitrogen or aerosol freezing solution (Histofreezer) may work. Some warts may require more than one treatment. Practice nurses can develop expertise in this field, but must be taught to perform the treatments safely. The hazards of cryotherapy include damage to tendons, nerves and joints. The wart or verruca should be pared with a scalpel before treatment but care is needed to avoid capillary bleeding. Children should only receive treatment if able to cooperate. Patients must be warned to expect blistering after the treatment and be told what to do and who to contact if advice is needed.

Insertion of intra-uterine device (IUD) or intra-uterine system (see Chapter 12)

The following sterile equipment is required:

- Cusco speculum
- long artery forceps
- sponge-holding forceps
- Volsellum forceps
- uterine sound
- Hagar's dilators
- long round-ended scissors
- gallipot and lotion
- disposal bag for clinical waste.

In addition sterile gloves, examination jelly, thread retriever, selection of IUDs, sanitary towel and the emergency tray will be required; glyceryl trinitrate spray, sterile local anaesthetic gel and an introducer may sometimes be required.

Unsterile demonstration IUDs are useful for teaching patients about the devices. A practice nurse needs to understand the insertion procedure in order to explain it to patients and to assist the practitioner when necessary.

The following procedure should be used:

(1) The patient should have an empty bladder and remove tights and pants; then be made comfortable on the couch and covered with a disposable paper sheet.
(2) The clinician may perform a bimanual examination, to identify any pelvic abnormalities.
(3) A vaginal speculum is inserted to visualise the cervix. The assistant may need to adjust the light.
(4) The cervix is cleaned with a swab moistened with a cleansing solution and held in the sponge-holding forceps.
(5) If the patient has an IUD in situ, it is removed with the long forceps and thread retriever if needed.

(6)   The tissue forceps may then be attached, to hold the cervix steady (not used by all clinicians).

(7)   The uterine sound is inserted through the cervix to assess the length and position of the uterine cavity.

(8)   The assistant opens the outer pack of the device selected and drops the contents onto the sterile field.

(9)   The clinician prepares the device and introducer and inserts it through the cervix into the uterine cavity. Sterile anaesthetic gel may be inserted to prevent pain and the dilators may be needed if there is a problem with insertion. The assistant may be asked to spray the GTN spray onto the cervix to make insertion easier.

(10)   Once inserted, the introducer is withdrawn, leaving the IUD or IUS in situ.

(11)   The threads are cut with the long scissors.

(12)   The speculum is removed.

(13)   The patient is allowed to rest until ready to dress.

On rare occasions, a patient may suffer cervical shock or a seizure; so the emergency equipment should be accessible. A patient with epilepsy could also have a seizure precipitated by the insertion of an IUD[13]. The nursing care of a patient having an IUD inserted is covered in Chapter 12 (Sexual health).

Suggestions for reflection on practice

- Review your most recent wound treatments in terms of healing, cost-effectiveness and patient satisfaction. What evidence supported the dressing choices?
- Review your practice policy and procedure for ear irrigation. Are any changes to procedure needed?
- Audit the outcomes of minor surgery. Did any patients have infections or healing problems afterwards? Are any changes to procedure needed?

Further reading

Harkin, H. & Vaz, F. (2001) Provision of ear care in the primary care setting. *Primary Health Care*, **10** (10), 30–33.

Hoggins, C. (2000) Cryosurgery in primary care. *Practice Nursing*, **11** (4), 21–3.

Lloyd-Jones, M. (2001) Wound cleansing. *Practice Nurse*, **22** (2), 22–6.

National Institute for Clinical Excellence (2001) *Guidance on the use of debriding agents and specialist wound care for difficult to heal wounds*. National Institute for Clinical Excellence, London.

Vickerstaff, E. (2001) Safe syringing. *Practice Nurse*, **21** (7), 24–8.

Watson, S. (2001) The pathophysiology of different types of leg ulcers. *British Journal of Community Nursing*, **6** (3), 118–24.

References

1. Parliament (1987) *The Consumer Protection Act 1987, Part 1 – Product Liability*. HMSO, London.
2. O'Sullivan, S.T., O'Connor, P. & O'Shaughnessy, M. (1996) Aetiology and management of hypertrophic scars and keloids. *Annals of Royal College of Surgeons of England*, **78**, 168–75.
3. Gilchrist, B. (1999) Wound infection. In *Wound Management Theory and Practice* (eds M. Miller & D. Glover). Nursing Times Books, London.
4. Winter, G. (1962) Formation of the scab and rate of epithelisation of superficial wounds in the skin of the young domestic pig. *Nature*, **193**, 293–4.
5. Ryatt, M. & Quinton, D. (1997) Tap water as a wound cleansing agent. *Journal of Accident and Emergency Nursing*, **14**, 165–6.
6. Lawton, S. (2001) Eczema. In: *Dermatology Nursing. A Practical Guide*. Churchill Livingstone, Edinburgh.
7. Siana, J. & Gottrup, F. (1992) The effects of smoking on tissue function. *Journal of Wound Care*, **1** (2), 37–41.
8. Eagle, M. (1999) Compression bandaging. *Nursing Standard*, **13** (20), 49–54.
9. Price, J. & Moss, J. (1998) The pitfalls of practice nursing. *Nursing Times*, **94** (30), 64–66.
10. British Medical Association, Royal Pharmaceutical Society of Great Britain (2001) *British National Formulary*, 41, 12.1.3. British Medical Association, Royal Pharmaceutical Society, London.
11. Rogers, R. (2000) Understand the legalities of ear syringing. *Practice Nurse*, **4** (19), 166–9.
12. Department of Health (2001) Risk assessment for transmission of vCJD via surgical instruments: a modelling approach and numerical scenarios. *www.doh.gov.uk/cjd/riskassessments* (accessed 18/8/01).
13. British Epilepsy Association (date unknown) Epilepsy and contraception. *Information – Epilepsy and Women*. *www.epilepsy.org.uk/info/epwomfrm.html* (accessed 5/9/01).

Useful addresses and web sites

Tissue Viability Society
Glanville Centre, Salisbury District Hospital, Salisbury SP2 8BJ
Web site: *www.tvs.org.uk*

Wound Care Society
PO Box 170, Hartford, Huntingdon PE29 1PL
Telephone/fax: 01480 434401
Web site: *www.woundcaresociety.org*

Biosurgical Research Unit (for LarvE maggots)
Bridgend, Glamorgan,
Telephone: 01656 75283 Fax: 01656 752830
Web site: *www.smtl.co.uk/WMPRC/Maggots*

Primary Ear Care Centre
Stag Medical Centre, 162 Wickersley Road, Rotherham S60 4JW
Telephone: 01709 835315

Centre for Innovation in Primary Care
www.innovate.org.uk

Chapter 6
Diagnostic and Screening Tests

A practice nurse may undertake a range of investigative and screening procedures, either self-initiated, or at the request of a GP. This will depend on local arrangements and guidelines and on the nurse's scope of professional practice. The standards for individual procedures should cover the following areas: nurse education, clinical guidelines, informed consent, health education, emergency procedures, records and management of specimens, and hand hygiene.

Nurse education

Some skills can be learned within the practice but for others training may be accessed through local trusts and teaching establishments. Expert tuition and practice under supervision are needed for cervical screening; in-house training is not recommended[1]. Accredited training in cervical screening is provided through Marie Curie and family planning courses, and postgraduate study. A practice nurse involved in taking cervical smears must have had the necessary theoretical and practical experience and be accountable for her practice. Whatever the test or investigation, the nurse owes a duty of care to his/her patients and must have the competence to perform the procedure satisfactorily through the appropriate training, supervision and updating. Any equipment used must be maintained and calibrated correctly.

Clinical guidelines

Many practice nurses are given the authority to test for rubella antibodies, serum lipids, glucose etc. There is a cost implication with most investigations and therefore decisions need to be made about who should be offered particular tests. Patients may self-refer for tests they have read about or discovered on the Internet, so guidelines are needed to cover such eventualities. The guidelines will specify when the practice nurse should refer on to another health professional. There will also need to be systems in place to react to test results, e.g. lipids and prostate-specific antigen. Some programmes for cervical cytology are run almost entirely by practice nurses.

Informed consent

Investigations must not be carried out without the patient's consent. Patients need accurate and detailed information and the opportunity to discuss possible implications of the results of the investigations to be performed[2]. Many tests can only be performed correctly if the patient knows what to expect and can cooperate. Tests for HIV antibodies must not be performed until the patient has been fully counselled and has decided to have the test[3]. Patients also need counselling about the test for prostate-specific antigen (see Chapter 14, Men's health).

Health education

Patients undergoing any sort of test are likely to be concerned about some aspect of their health. Most situations, if sensitively handled, present a chance for health promotion. For example, patients frequently express half-joking hopes that clean equipment is being used. Such expressions of concern offer a way of openly discussing worries about blood-borne virus (BBV) infection. The prevention of coronary heart disease is part of the nurse's health promotion role. A patient attending for an ECG, even for medical insurance purposes, is likely to be interested in his/her health, so a discussion of the lifestyle factors likely to affect the heart may sometimes be appropriate.

Emergency procedures

Familiarity is needed with the local guidelines for dealing with needlestick injuries, splashes or spillages of blood or body fluids, and for coping with a patient who collapses for any reason.

Records and management of specimens

Good record keeping is an important tool in promoting high quality health care[4]. Pathology forms must be completed accurately and the specimen containers labelled with the correct identification details. Details of foreign travel, fasting, medication or last menstrual period may be needed for specific tests. Failure to provide such details can affect the interpretation of the results. The practice requires a foolproof system for recording specimens sent for testing and results received. Samples should be placed in sealed specimen bags before despatch to the laboratory. The Post Office has regulations requiring the secure packaging of any specimens sent by post[5]. Biohazard stickers may still be requested by laboratory staff on specimen bottles and forms of patients known to pose a high risk of infectious diseases such as hepatitis B, although in reality all specimens should be considered as potentially hazardous and be handled accordingly.

The laboratory should be consulted if there is doubt about a specimen that cannot be despatched the same day. Some tests give false results if delayed. Urine can be kept in a refrigerator at 4°C overnight. This delay should be noted on the form. Swabs in transport medium can be kept in a cool place but should not be put in the fridge. Some blood samples ought not to be refrigerated. If in doubt, guidance can be sought from the laboratory on the storage of specimens awaiting collection.

All tests and their results must be entered in the patients' records. The patient must know how he/she will be notified of the result(s). Some investigations take longer than others, so a patient required to telephone for results needs to know how many tests were performed and when the results are likely to be available. The electronic transfer of laboratory results is becoming ever more common and can save time and assist in the provision of a more reliable service. However, the use of computers will not prevent problems if the system for checking and acting on abnormal results is not robust.

Hand hygiene

Hand washing will not be mentioned in any of the procedures given below because it is taken for granted that qualified nurses are aware of this most important method of preventing cross-infection and will automatically wash their hands before and after hand contact with patients. Gloves should be worn whenever necessary.

Laboratory tests

A good relationship with the local laboratory staff is worth cultivating. Most pathology departments will supply a list of tests; giving the amounts of sample material needed, the type of specimen bottle and any special requirements, such as timing or diet.

Blood tests

Requirements

The following equipment is required:

- vacuum system needles and holders
- sample tubes and pathology forms including plastic bag
- arm cushion with protective cover
- tourniquet and/or sphygmomanometer and cuff
- powder free unsterile latex gloves (alternative if allergy to latex)
- alcohol wipes and cotton wool balls or gauze swabs
- small adhesive plasters/hypoallergenic tape
- sharps container and yellow clinical waste bag.

Vacuum systems are considered to be safer because blood is drawn directly into the specimen bottles thus reducing the risk of nurse contact with the patient's blood. Different sizes of double-ended needles are available and the appropriate size should be selected for each patient. Disposable holders are available but in some areas, reusable holders are used in conjunction with a device for removing the needles. If in doubt about the safety of a system, nurses are advised to consult the local infection control nurse for guidance.

Venepuncture

The following procedure should be followed:

Action	Rationale
Approach the patient confidently and explain the procedure	To explain the tests, to reduce anxiety and to obtain the patient's cooperation and consent
Consult the patient regarding any previously identified problems; the patient should be allowed time to discuss these	To involve the patient in his or her treatment; to identify any factors that may influence vein choice
Offer an anxious patient the opportunity to lie down while blood is taken *or* seat the patient where the arm can be supported; use a small arm pillow if needed	Recumbent patients will be less likely to faint and can be managed more easily if they do
Verify that all identification details on the request form are correct, gather specimen tubes and required equipment and place equipment close enough so all is within easy reach	To ensure that the appropriate samples are taken from the correct patient
Ask the patient to roll up his/her sleeve or ask to remove the arm from the garment if too tight	To make sure the vein can be accessed easily (tight clothing above the elbow can contribute to haematoma formation)
Attach the double-ended needle to the holder	Vacuum sample tubes can be attached once the needle is in the vein
Apply the tourniquet above the elbow Remember, most patients have two arms so make sure the best site is selected	To distend the vein in the antecubital fossa There can be marked difference between the arms in the accessibility of veins
Cleanse the skin with the alcohol wipe and wait for the alcohol to dry	To remove bacteria from the skin and avoid stinging at the puncture site
Insert the needle at an appropriate angle and keep it still once in situ	Depending on the depth of the vein (too steep an angle might cause the needle tip to pass right through the vein)

(Continued)

Action (continued)	Rationale (continued)
Attach each vacuum tube in turn, keeping the needle steady while doing so	Depending on the type of samples needed and to avoid trauma to the vein wall

Attach tubes in the order:
   plain tubes
   tubes with anticoagulants
   other tubes with additives
Note: the tourniquet should be released before collecting blood for calcium levels or lipids
	To reduce the chance of contamination of clotted samples by anticoagulant or other additives

Gently invert the tubes upon removal	To mix the blood with the anticoagulant etc. (not necessary if clotted samples are needed)
Release the tourniquet	To release the pressure on the vein
Remove the needle and holder, apply a cotton wool ball or swab over the puncture site and ask the patient to apply pressure for one or two minutes with the arm straight	Extravasion of the blood at the puncture site can cause bruising or a haematoma (particular care is needed with patients on warfarin or with abnormal liver function, who may bleed for longer)
Dispose of the needle and disposable holder in a sharps bin	To avoid the danger of needlestick injury
Cover the puncture site with a small sterile adhesive plaster or bandage if necessary	To prevent infection (use a bandage if allergic to adhesives or prolonged bleeding likely)
Ensure that the pathology form and sample tubes have all the correct details	Unlabelled specimens will not be processed, biochemistry samples with the wrong date may be rejected
Make sure the patient knows when and how to get the test results	

If a syringe and needle is used:

(1) Select a syringe large enough to fill all the sample bottles needed.
(2) Withdraw the blood steadily, using gentle traction on the piston because too fast an action may haemolyse the cells but too slow a collection may allow the blood to coagulate.
(3) Squirting blood through the needle can damage the cells and affect some test results, especially electrolytes. Either allow the vacuum in the tube to draw the blood in, or if necessary, remove the needle from the syringe and the cap from the tube and gently fill the tube from the syringe. Replace the lid on the sample tube with care.
(4) Fill the sample tubes to the required level because precise quantities of blood may be needed for some tests, such as ESR and coagulation tests.

In the event of accidental blood spillage, splash or needlestick injury follow the practice procedure (see Chapter 4).

Urine tests

Urine for microbiology

Midstream specimen of urine (MSU) This test is meant to identify any organisms causing infection inside the urinary tract. Hence the need to collect specimens which are uncontaminated by skin and perineal flora. The genital area should be washed and a specimen obtained after the urine flow has started. A sterile receptacle can be used if the patient cannot pass the specimen directly into the sample container. Discussing the collection of an MSU may also provide an opportunity to educate the patient about urinary tract infections and ways of preventing reinfection.

Clean catch specimen of urine When a midstream urine specimen cannot be obtained, or is not necessary, the urine can be voided into a clean container. Special collection bags with an adhesive flange can be attached to the genital area of infants. The bags are expensive, but small quantities can be purchased from medical supply firms. However, many laboratories will ask for a clean catch specimen from children under two years. This is because of the high number of contaminated specimens collected in bags[6].

Urine for cytology Malignant cells in the urinary tract can be detected in urine samples. The patient should be instructed to void most of the urine and collect the sample (10–20 ml) towards the end of the stream.

First-catch urine for Chlamydia This may be a more acceptable *Chlamydia* test for the patient, which can give reliable results[7]. The availability of urine tests for *Chlamydia* will depend on the facilities of the local laboratory. If a urine specimen for *Chlamydia* is requested, the patient should be asked not to pass urine for at least one hour. Then the first 20 ml of urine should be collected in a sterile universal container.

24-hour urine collections Large plastic containers and instruction sheets for collecting 24-hour specimens can be obtained from the laboratory. The containers for VMA analysis contain acid as a preservative and need safe storage. Dietary restrictions are needed before some tests. The patient should pass urine normally at the time of starting the collection and then save all the urine passed over the next 24 hours, finishing at the same time next day. A clotted blood sample may also be requested for serum creatinine if 24-hour urine is collected for creatinine clearance.

Cervical smears
(see Chapter 13, Women's health)

There is a national call and recall system for all women aged 20–64 years of age in the United Kingdom. Practices have to reach a target of 80% or a lower target of 50% of eligible women screened in order to qualify for payments for cervical screening. The success of cervical screening depends on two factors:

- ensuring that women attend for screening
- obtaining adequate smears.

Practice nurses can help on both counts; by educating women about the need for screening, by facilitating access to the service and by learning to take good smears gently and sympathetically. Interpreting services may be needed when patients do not understand English and may not have had experience of cervical screening. Education in cultural awareness can have particular significance when dealing with this intimate procedure.

Note: smear-taking cannot be learned from a book; the following is only intended as a reminder.

Requirements

The following are required:

- couch and good, adjustable, heat-filtered light
- unsterile examination gloves
- glass microscope slide and pencil
- vaginal specula in range of sizes
- KY jelly
- Aylesbury spatula, and cervical brush (or according to protocol)
- fixing tray
- carbowax fixative
- tissues
- slide carrier
- cytology request form.

Procedure

The following procedure should be used:

Action	Rationale
Explain the procedure and answer any questions	To obtain consent and to make sure the patient knows what to expect
Check the details with the patient and complete the cytology form	To provide the cytologist with all the relevant information for interpreting the slide and notifying the patient of the result

(Continued)

Action (continued)	*Rationale (continued)*
Note the date of the last menstrual period	The microscopic appearance of cells varies during the cycle, with hormonal influences
Enquire about any discharge, abnormal bleeding or pain	Further investigations or medical examination may be needed
Write the patient's name and date of birth on the opaque end of the glass slide	For identification and correlation with the pathology form
Ensure the room is warm, privacy is guaranteed and the patient has emptied her bladder	To help her relax and be comfortable during the procedure
Ask the patient to remove her undergarments and lie on the couch	To allow a clear view of the genital area
Place the speculum in warm water (body temperature)	To warm and lubricate the instrument and thus to avoid discomfort for the patient
Position the patient with her knees bent and legs apart, or in left lateral position, adjust the light	To ensure a good view can be obtained of the vulva and cervix
Put on examination gloves	
Observe the vulva for any lesions, bleeding, discharge or soreness	To detect any abnormalities or signs of infection or disease
Remove excess water from the speculum, use a small amount of lubricant only if needed	Water can macerate the cells and excess lubricant may affect the quality of the cell sample
Part the labia and insert the closed speculum halfway into the vagina. Turn the speculum, gently manoeuvre it and open the blades	To view the cervix
Withdraw the speculum if unable to visualise the cervix: digital vaginal examination may be necessary; a different speculum or patient position may be needed	To locate the cervix manually before a second attempt
Note the condition of the cervix	To detect any problems, e.g. prolapse, polyps, warts, discharge or abnormal appearance
Pass the tip of the spatula through the speculum and with the longest part resting in the cervical os, turn the spatula through a full circle twice, using pencil-writing pressure (widen the circle of turn if an ectropion is noted)	To obtain cells from the transformation zone – the junction of squamous and columnar cells where pre-malignant cells are most likely to be located The position of the squamo-columnar junction can vary with age
Take a second sample with a cervical brush if appropriate	According to the local guidelines

(Continued)

Action (continued)	Rationale (continued)
Spread the sample material onto the glass slide, using two long strokes for each side of the spatula, covering half the clear surface of the slide each time	To provide a satisfactory cell sample and avoid damaging the cells
Roll the brush, if used, along the clear surface of a separate slide marked with the patient's details	A second slide should be used for a brush sample and must be marked accordingly to inform the cytological examiner
Hold the fixative bottle with a tissue or with the turned back sleeve of the glove	To avoid contaminating the fixative bottle
Place the slide(s) flat in a purpose-made fixing tray or across two pencils; flood the slide(s) with the fixative and leave them to dry	To preserve the cells on the slide
Remove the vaginal speculum, noting the condition of the vaginal walls in the process	Some experienced nurses may remove the speculum before fixing the slide but there is a danger of unfixed material drying if left too long
Place the speculum in a receiver containing water	To assist cleaning by preventing the drying of secretions on the speculum
Invite the patient to get dressed, if a vaginal examination is not needed	Pelvic examination is not recommended for asymptomatic patients[9] (the practice procedure should indicate the action to be taken if a patient reports abnormal symptoms)
Record any pertinent details on the cytology form	To inform the cytologist of any technical problems or observations of the condition of the cervix
Once dried, place the slide in a slide box	To prevent accidental breakage and for safe transport of the slide to the laboratory

The patient needs to know how she will be notified of the result and to understand the significance of any result.

Problems with inserting the speculum should alert the nurse to possible sexual difficulties that the patient may be encountering. Involuntary contraction of the vaginal wall muscles (vaginismus) can prevent penetration. Sensitive questions about problems with intercourse can be asked and referral made to the appropriate source of help and advice if the patient needs more help than the nurse feels competent to provide.

Swabs

Samples of infected material can be obtained from any accessible part of the body by using a sterile swab stick tipped with cotton wool or synthetic material. Commercially produced swabs are packaged with plastic tubes for transport. Once the patient has understood and agreed to the procedure, the swab should be gently rotated in the material for culture and transferred immediately to the container. Swabs are available for both bacterial and viral culture and for *Chlamydia* DNA.

Nasal swabs   Moisten the swab with sterile saline solution because the mucosa is usually dry. Organisms will adhere more easily to a moist swab. Rotate the tip of the swab inside the anterior nares. Per nasal swabs may occasionally be needed. Contact the local laboratory for details.

Throat swabs   A good light is required to visualise the throat. A tongue depressor may be needed to see the throat and prevent contamination of the sample if swabbing stimulates the gag reflex. Take the swab from the tonsil area or any exudate.

Ear swabs   Rotate the swab tip gently at the entrance of the auditory meatus before any treatment drops are used. This will prevent infecting organisms being masked by the treatment drops.

Vaginal swabs   Gently part the labia to visualise the introitus and swab inside the vagina.

High vaginal swabs   Pass a speculum (as described for taking cervical smears) to visualise the cervix. Swab the discharge in the posterior fornix and withdraw the swab carefully, avoiding contact with the vaginal walls and vulva.

Endocervical swabs   The cervix is first cleaned with a large-headed cotton wool swab, if provided (according to local policy). The endocervical swab is rotated in the endocervix for 30 seconds, to obtain the specimen. A sample of cells is needed to test for *Chlamydia* DNA, unlike the samples of discharge collected by other swabs. The sample must immediately be placed in the transport container and be stored and transported in accordance with the manufacturer's instructions[9].

Urethral swabs   Retract the prepuce of an uncircumcised male patient, or part the labia if a female. Swab the urethral orifice.

Rectal swabs   Gently pass the tip of the swab through the anus into the rectum. Rotate the swab and withdraw it. *Chlamydia* testing may be needed sometimes. Referral to a GU clinic is recommended.

Skin and nail samples

Skin scrapings or clippings may be sent to the laboratory in a commercial mycological pack (these may be available from the laboratory, drug companies or purchased from medical suppliers). A sufficient sample for testing is required for microscopy and culture[10].

Threadworms

Threadworms lay their eggs outside the anus at night. Either swab the perianal area to detect threadworm ova or alternatively, instruct the patient/parent to use a piece of clear adhesive tape next to the anus, to collect the sample. Seal the tape onto a ground glass slide for microscopy.

Faeces

Specimens of faeces are usually collected by the patient at home, in a special container with a spoon attached. Instruct the patient to empty his/her bladder and then place about six layers of toilet paper into the toilet pan, pass the stool onto the paper and scoop a small section of the stool into the container with the spoon provided. Alternatively the patient should place a sheet of cling film across the toilet pan beneath the seat (not tightly!). Pass the stool, collect the specimen as before, release the cling film and flush away. The importance of hand washing should be stressed. Samples for microbiology must be taken directly to the laboratory. Consult the laboratory about special instructions for stool specimens for occult blood or faecal fat.

Practice nurses can provide information on basic hygiene and food handling to all patients with diarrhoea. Professional food handlers with gastrointestinal infections must be clear of infection before returning to work.

Semen

Patients may be required to produce semen samples for infertility investigations, to check the effectiveness of vasectomy operations, or other urological tests. The sample of ejaculate should be collected in a sterile, wide specimen container and taken to the laboratory immediately, in accordance with local guidelines.

Sputum

Sputum specimens can be requested for microbiology or cytology. The patient should be given a wide sterile specimen container and asked to produce a specimen of sputum after some deep productive coughing; preferably in the morning before eating or drinking. The physiotherapist may be asked to help patients who are unable to expectorate. Nebulised normal saline can also be used to aid expectoration.

Investigations and tests within the practice

Blood tests

Tests performed on site allow the results to be available more quickly.

Blood glucose

Commercially produced test strips and meters give accurate results providing a few simple rules are followed:

- Always follow the manufacturer's instructions
- Follow the instructions for quality control and keep records of control tests
- Keep the test strips dry in sealed containers
- Discard out-of-date strips
- Use a drop of blood large enough to cover the test area
- Make sure the meter is calibrated to match the strips
- Keep the meter clean and renew the battery when necessary
- Record results immediately.

An automatic device makes the finger prick less painful by controlling the depth and speed of the puncture. A disposable lancet must be used for each patient.

Erythrocyte sedimentation rate (ESR)

ESR is a measure of how fast the red cells collect as sediment in a vertical tube. It is a non-specific test to indicate the presence or absence of inflammatory processes. Blood can be sent to the laboratory, or the test may be performed in the surgery, using either a disposable, plastic, calibrated tube, or more usually, a vacuum-system, glass tube in a special stand. The test should be set up according to the manufacturer's instructions and the level of sedimentation noted after one hour. An automatic timer can help to ensure a reading is not forgotten. After an hour the sedimentation rate becomes more rapid, so can give a falsely high reading. The normal ESR range is 3–10 mm/hr for men and 5–15 mm/hr for women, although measurements just above the range are common and need to be interpreted carefully. Normal readings may be higher for patients over 50 years old – up to 20 mm/hr for men and 30 mm/hr for women.

Clinical chemistry analysis

Compact microprocessor instruments are already available for performing a range of blood tests on site. Results can be printed out for the patients' records. The advantages of near-patient tests, such as INR, HbA_{1c} or lipids, include the saving of time and reduced number of visits for patients, as well as allowing the immediacy of treatment. Disadvantages include the costs of purchasing and maintaining the machines as well as the need for robust quality control measures to ensure their accuracy at all times.

Urine tests

A range of diptests are available for urinalysis. They have a limited shelf-life once opened and some are very costly. It pays to select the most suitable product for the tests required because most have to be purchased by the practice. Some combination strips are available in smaller quantities, more suitable for use in general practice. Single type test strips, e.g. for glucose, albumin and ketones are prescribable for individual patients. All test strips must be kept dry, with the bottle top replaced immediately after use. The desiccant sachet must not be removed. The type of test done should be specified when recording results. Urine specimens should be emptied into a toilet rather than a sink.

Pregnancy tests

Pregnancy tests can be bought in bulk. They detect human chorionic gonadotrophic hormone excreted in urine by pregnant women. Hence the usual requirement for testing the first specimen of the day – early morning urine (EMU), when the urine is most concentrated. The tests give a result within minutes and are easy to use. The manufacturer's instructions should be followed. The tests are expensive and have to be purchased by the practice, so a policy is needed about using them. Patients can buy their own tests from a pharmacy and if a patient has already had a positive home test, there is usually little point in repeating it. However, not all patients can afford the expense of a home test. Patients who request tests too frequently may have other concerns about contraception and need help or advice.

The practice should also have a policy for documenting that patients have received the result of their pregnancy tests. As a salutary tale note the following: a patient, who had a miscarriage abroad, subsequently denied that she had been told she was pregnant and tried to blame the GP practice. The practice nurse knew that she had spoken to the patient on the telephone and had discussed the advisability of going on holiday but was unable to prove it because she had not documented the conversation.

Microscopy

The use of a microscope is mainly limited to looking for pus cells in urine when a urinary tract infection is suspected. Although other uses include looking for fungal hyphae in nail or skin scrapings, *Trichomonas vaginalis* in vaginal discharge, or for looking at blood smears. The degree of microscope use might depend on the accessibility of a pathology laboratory but it could provide the opportunity to commence treatment before laboratory results are available.

Electrocardiography

The ECG records electrical potential in the heart muscle as it beats. The various electrical pathways are altered in muscle which has been damaged or where the heart is beating irregularly. These changes give the tracing its characteristic appearance and assist in the diagnosis of cardiac problems. A patient may be asked to exercise under supervision before, or as, the recording is made. This could be dangerous in the absence of full resuscitation equipment and appropriately trained staff, so exercise ECGs are usually performed in hospital. Machines vary, so the maker's instruction must be followed. Nurses who have not worked in coronary care require training in the recording and interpretation of ECGs.

Requirements

The following will be required:

- ECG machine
- disposable electrode patches or reusable electrodes with contact jelly/cream
- alcohol skin wipes
- unused disposable razor
- ballpoint pen.

Procedure

The following procedure should be used:

Action	Rationale
Ensure privacy and a warm room temperature	The patient will need to undress and shivering will affect the recording
Make sure the patient knows what to expect and that it will be painless	The wires can look like something from a horror movie and cause unnecessary anxiety
Ask the patient to undress as needed	The chest, arms and ankles will need to be accessible
Assist him/her onto the couch and make as comfortable as possible	So he/she can lie still during the procedure
Apply the electrode to the wrists, ankles and chest (if the skin is greasy use the alcohol wipes; very hairy skin may need to be shaved in order to get skin contact)	To create a good contact between the skin and the electrodes in order to detect the electrical activity as the heart muscle contracts and relaxes
Attach the correct wires to the electrodes	
Begin the recording when the patient is relaxed	Movement will cause electrical interference
If the machine does not automatically record all the required tracings, follow the maker's instructions for recording leads I, II, III, AVR, AVL, AVF and the six V leads in turn	To record the electrical potential from different directions

(Continued)

Action (continued)	Rationale (continued)
Record approximately five complexes per tracing, if not done automatically	Adequate for interpretation without wasting recording paper
Record another longer tracing of II (10–12 complexes), if not done automatically	To act as a rhythm strip (lead II is usually closest to the cardiac vector – the direction and strength of electrical voltage of the heart as it contracts)
If not automatically marked by the machine, mark each trace with the ballpoint pen	To help the reader to identify each tracing and compare it with the norm
Make sure the patient's name, date of birth and date of recording is on the ECG sheet	For filing and comparison with previous recordings

If there is interference with the ECG tracing:

- There may be interference from other electrical equipment or the metal frame of the couch
- Check the electrodes are giving good skin contact
- Check the wires are attached to the correct electrodes
- Check that the machine is on the correct settings if automatic
- The machine may need servicing.

When all the tracings have been taken satisfactorily remove the electrodes, wipe any contact jelly/cream off the skin and invite the patient to get dressed.

Interpreting results   Nurses who perform electrocardiography must be able to recognise an abnormal tracing so that the appropriate actions, in accordance with the practice guidelines, can be taken before the patient leaves the surgery.

Respiratory function tests

Peak expiratory flow rate (PEFR)

Peak flow meters measure the amount of air that a patient is capable of expelling forcibly from the lungs. It is not the volume of air that is measured, but the rate of expulsion. This is directly related to the elasticity of the lungs and the volume of air within the lungs, and is measured in litres expelled per minute. The normal range for an adult male of about 1.80 m in height would be 550–700 l/min. The normal varies according to height, sex and age. Tables are available to give guidance on this. These guides constitute the predicted levels against which an individual patient's results can be compared.

   Use of a peak flow meter is vital to the modern treatment of asthma. Indeed many patients with asthma are encouraged to keep one at home and use it regularly. A fall in the peak flow rate may be the first indication of the onset of severe asthma (see Chapter 7 under emergency treatment of asthma, and Chapter 16 under asthma management). The modern equivalent of the Wright's peak flow meter, the Mini-Wright's meter, is a small plastic tube with a scale along the top and a moveable indicator. This type, and similar meters, can be prescribed on FP10. Low range peak flow meters are available for children.

Measuring peak expiratory flow rate   This is done in the following way:

Action	Rationale
Ask the patient to stand up	To allow the maximum expansion of the chest
Ask the patient to hold the meter horizontally and to keep the fingers away from the indicator, which must be set at zero	To allow the indicator to move freely along the scale
Then to take a deep slow breath, place the lips around the mouthpiece and breathe out as quickly and forcibly as possible	To expand the lungs fully and then exhale as quickly as possible into the PEF meter

If the procedure has been performed correctly, or the patient is not too breathless, the indicator will move along the scale and the reading can be taken. The whole manoeuvre can then be repeated two more times, if possible, and the best of the three readings recorded and compared with the predicted level for the patient's age and height. Forced expiration can make a patient feel dizzy so they should be observed carefully throughout the procedure. Patients can be taught to plot their home PEFR readings in a Peak Flow Diary.

Spirometry

Many practices now own a spirometer for measuring lung function. The manufacturer's instructions for the use of the instrument should be followed and training in spirometry is absolutely essential (see Chapter 16 under COPD).
   A spirometer can record:

- The vital capacity – the total amount exhaled normally after a maximum inhalation
- The forced expiratory volume (FEV_1) – the amount that can be forcibly breathed out in one second following a maximum inhalation
- The forced vital capacity (FVC) – the amount of air forcibly exhaled after a maximum inhalation.

The results can be read from the liquid crystal display (or through an attached computer) and compared with predicted levels. Comparisons of the actual recordings with the predicted results for each patient can demonstrate the existence and severity of obstructive pulmonary disease or restrictive airways disease. A calculator would usually be needed to calculate the results for a hand-held spirometer.

Respiratory function tests may also be used in health screening by demonstrating to smokers any existing lung damage and the benefits of quitting the habit.

Patients who are pregnant, have recently undergone surgery (especially ENT or eye surgery) or have a history of pneumothorax should not undertake forced expiratory tests[11].

Preparation of the patient   Before carrying out the test prepare the patient in the following way:

- If possible, bronchodilator drugs should not be used for six hours before the test
- Non-restrictive clothing should be worn
- The patient should have an empty bladder, especially if prone to stress incontinence.

Procedure   Follow the procedure below:

Action	Rationale
Seat the patient comfortably in an upright position	The procedure can cause dizziness or faintness so the patient should not be standing
Explain and demonstrate the technique	To get the patient's consent and ensure the test is performed correctly
Ask the patient to breathe in as deeply as possible, to seal the lips around the mouthpiece and exhale slowly and completely	To determine the relaxed vital capacity (the nurse may need to press the start button on the machine as the patient begins the exhalation)
Repeat the procedure and record the best of the two results	
Repeat the procedure but this time ask the patient to breathe out forcibly for as long as possible and encourage the patient not to stop too soon	To determine the forced vital capacity and FEV_1 (this is a different procedure from peak flow measurement)
Ask the patient to repeat the procedure at least two more times (but not more than five more times); allow time to recover the breath in between	Three readings should be similar (good reproducibility)
Record the best results for FVC and FEV_1, as well as the patient's age, height and gender	For comparison with the predicted levels and assessment of lung function

False results will be obtained if the patient:

- Starts exhaling too slowly
- Does not inhale and exhale fully
- Stops blowing into the spirometer too soon
- Coughs during the procedure
- Takes another breath in while performing the test.

Screening audiometry

Hearing tests for young children are either undertaken by health visitors or at hearing clinics. Other patients suspected of hearing loss may be referred to the practice nurse for a screening audiogram. This procedure will usually indicate in adults, and children old enough to participate, a hearing problem that requires further investigation. A history should be noted of any ear infections or injuries, speech or learning difficulties, or family history of deafness. The ears should be examined and the test postponed until any problems such as impacted wax or infection have been treated.

A screening audiogram entails recording the quietest sound the patient can hear in a range of frequencies (usually between 500 and 8000 hertz), working down in 5–10 decibel steps from 60 or 30 dB. A quiet room is needed for the test. Distractions must be avoided as concentration may be lost. Children must be old enough to understand what is required and be able to cooperate. The machine must be checked before use and be serviced and re-calibrated annually. A record should be kept of the service date. Children will get bored if the test is prolonged. If it is apparent that a patient, particularly a child, is responding inappropriately, the test should be discontinued and arrangements made for referral to the audiometry outpatients department. In some areas ENT consultants are not in favour of screening audiometry in general practice, but where it is performed, the results need to be interpreted correctly. If there is obvious hearing loss or an equivocal result, the patient should be referred. Some machines print out the results, but if not they can be plotted by hand. It may be helpful to show patients some examples in graph form of normal and impaired hearing. Some patients might benefit from using a hearing aid. It is better to learn to use them while young enough to adapt. Practice nurses can encourage patients to persevere with their aids to prevent social isolation in later life.

Vision testing

Visual acuity is tested by reading letters of decreasing size at a measured distance from a Snellen chart. Special charts are available for patients who are illiterate or too young to read. The Snellen chart should be attached to the wall and be well illuminated. A patient who normally wears spectacles for distance vision should be tested with the glasses on, with this noted on the record.

Visual acuity testing

Action	Rationale
Measure six meters from the chart and ask the patient to stand at the six-meter mark	The chart is designed to be read at this distance
Ask the patient to cover one eye gently	Each eye is tested in turn
Ask the patient to read the letters on the chart, starting from the top	To discover the smallest letters which can be read correctly
Record the number of the last complete line to be read accurately	Each line is marked with the distance at which it can be read by a normal eye
Repeat the procedure with the other eye	

The largest letter can be read by a person with normal sight from 60 meters, and the smallest letters from four meters. The result of a person reading from six meters distance who can read the sixth line (9 m) is written as 6/9. The test result of a patient with poor vision who can only see the top line is written as 6/60.

Patients who cannot see any of the letters on the chart may be tested to see if they can identify hand movements, or are able to perceive light.

Suggestions for reflection on practice

- Consider your role in dealing with tests and investigations.
- Could some of the work be delegated?
- Could the service to patients be improved in any way?

Further reading

NHS (1996) *Cervical Screening – A Pocket Guide*. Sheffield NHS Cervical Screening Programme.

Wolfenden, M. (Revised 1995) *Taking Cervical Smears*. British Society for Cervical Cytology, Orpington.

References

1. Department of Health (1998) *Cervical Screening Action Team – The Report*, Para. 20. Department of Health, London.
2. BMA (2001) Bristol Royal Infirmary Inquiry briefing papers, Briefing note on Consent and Risk. British Medical Association Public Affairs Division, London.

3. World Health Organisation (1993) Factsheet 7, *Counselling and HIV/Aids*. World Health Organisation, Geneva.

4. United Kingdom Central Council for Nurses, Midwives and Health Visitors (1998) *Guidelines for Records and Record Keeping*. UKCC, London.

5. Royal Mail (1994) *Prohibited and Restricted Goods: a few limitations on goods that may be sent from main Post*. Royal Mail Customer Services.

6. Cox, C. (2001) *Laboratory Diagnoses of Paediatric Urinary Tract Infection in the Under Twos* (Microbiology), *Follow-up: Monitoring implementation of project recommendations, Specialist Clinical Audit Programme*. Brighton and Hove Health Authority, East Sussex.

7. Bandolier (1998) *Chlamydia. www.jr2.ox.ac.uk/bandolier/band51/b51–2* (accessed 5/9/01).

8. Austoker, J. (1994) Cancer prevention in primary care: Screening for ovarian, prostatic and testicular cancers. *British Medical Journal*, **309** (6950), 315.

9. Grun, L. Tassano-Smith, J. Carder, C. *et al*. (1997) Comparison of two methods of screening for genital chlamydial infection in women attending in general practice: cross sectional survey, *British Medical Journal*, **315** (7102), 226–30.

10. Denning, D. Evans, E., Kibbler, C. *et al*. (1995) Fungal nail disease: a guide to good practice (report of a Working Group of the British Society for Medical Mycology) *British Medical Journal*, **311** (7015), 1277–81.

11. National Asthma and Respiratory Training Centre (2001) Spirometry Essential Skills Workshop. National Asthma and Respiratory Training Centre, Warwick.

Chapter 7
Emergency Situations

From time to time life-threatening crises will occur in the practice. Moreover, a practice nurse will sometimes be the only professionally qualified member of staff on the premises when an emergency call is received. He/she may be expected to assess the degree of urgency of the request and to decide on the appropriate course of action. Thorough training in emergency procedures and regular updates are needed for all the front line staff. The fact that the skills are called upon so rarely makes it even more vital to have regular practice sessions.

Accidents by their very nature, happen without warning, but many of them could be anticipated and prevented. One of the objectives in *Saving Lives: Our Healthier Nation* is a reduction of the death rate caused by accidents by at least a fifth and serious injury by at least a tenth by the year 2010[1]. So, apart from dealing with any emergencies which occur, medical and nursing staff also have a role in educating patients about safety.

General principles

While a practice nurse is unlikely to encounter situations involving multiple casualties, nevertheless he/she must always be aware that these could happen and first aid skills need to be kept up to date. The following general principles always apply:

Action	Rationale
Check that it is safe to approach the casualty	To avoid putting self or others in danger
Maintain a calm manner and take charge confidently	To prevent panic and to resist the pressure to act in haste
Collect as much relevant information as possible	To decide on the priorities for action
Deal with life-threatening emergencies immediately	To maintain the patient's respiration and circulation
Arrange for medical help from the GP or ambulance service if necessary	(Depending on the severity of the problem)

Whether giving advice over the telephone, rendering first aid at the site of an accident, or dealing with an incident in the surgery, three factors have priority:

A – Airway – must be clear for air entry to the lungs
B – Breathing – must be present to oxygenate the blood
C – Circulation – is essential for perfusion of the brain and vital organs[2].

Collapse

Any sudden prostration or loss of consciousness is loosely termed *collapse*. The reason may be obvious when it happens in the surgery, but on other occasions an assessment of all the clues will be needed. The action to be taken will depend on the cause of the collapse and the age of the patient. Any of the following scenarios could apply. Consult the *Resuscitation Guidelines 2000*[3]. The Resuscitation Council UK guidelines are updated regularly in line with medical evidence. Copies of the most recent guidelines can be obtained via the Internet or by post.

Collapsed but conscious patient

Check it is safe to approach. Attempt to rouse the patient. Does the patient respond to calling or a gentle shake of the shoulders? Avoid shaking infants because of the risk of brain damage. Shaking of any patient should be avoided if a neck injury is a possibility. If the patent is conscious then obtain information about his/her condition, treat as appropriate and summon help if needed. Continue regular reassessments.

Collapsed unconscious patient

Check as above (for collapsed but conscious patient). If there is no response call for help then follow the ABC:

Airway

- Check that the upper airway is clear. Leave well-fitting dentures in place but clear the mouth of any obvious obstruction. Blind finger sweeps of the mouth of a child should be avoided because they could cause swelling of the soft tissues or further impaction of a foreign body.
- Tilt the patient's head backwards and lift the patient's lower jaw without moving the neck. Use one finger under the chin and avoid pressing under the jaw of a child because pressure on the soft tissues can obstruct the airway.

Breathing

- Check if the patient is breathing by looking at the chest for signs of movement, listening for breath sounds and feeling for expired air against your cheek (for no more than ten seconds)

- If normal breathing is present turn the patient into the recovery position, send or go for help and continue to reassess the breathing about once a minute.
- If the patient is not breathing or is making only occasional gasps follow the adult or paediatric resuscitation guidelines as appropriate. Up to five attempts should be made to give two effective breaths.

Circulation

- Check the carotid pulse if the patient is over one year old (or the brachial pulse if an infant), for no more than ten seconds. (People with no healthcare training are no longer expected to try and locate a pulse.)
- If confident the patient has a circulation then continue rescue breathing as necessary and reassess about once a minute.
- Move the patient into the recovery position if spontaneous breathing occurs. Continue to reassess.
- If a circulation is not detected or unsure about a circulation start chest compressions. If the heart rate is less than 60 beats/minute in a child also start chest compressions.

Rescue breathing   If rescue breathing is taking place in the practice, a resuscitation mask with a one-way valve would normally be used, but it is essential to have had recent practice in using a mask effectively. This applies equally to the use of a reservoir bag and mask. A mask will cover both the patient's mouth and the nose. If the mask has an oxygen attachment then 100% oxygen should be used. The Basic Life Support guidelines attempt to deal with any eventuality and therefore the procedure will need to be adapted when using resuscitation equipment. The patient's mouth needs to be clear from obstruction and a clear airway position maintained.

The adult procedure is as follows:

- Pinch the patient's nose to close the nostrils.
- Open his/her mouth slightly but maintain the chin lift.
- Take a deep breath, close your mouth around the patient's mouth to obtain a good seal and blow steadily into his/her mouth for about two seconds. There should be only minimal resistance.
- Turn your face sideways and watch the patient's chest fall.
- Take another breath and repeat the sequence to give two effective breaths.

The paediatric procedure is as follows:

- Children – as for an adult but use only as much air as is necessary to inflate the chest. Blow for one to one and a half seconds. Repeat up to five times to ensure two effective breaths achieved.
- Infants – as for a child but breathe into the nose and mouth of a small infant, or the nose alone of an older one. If the nose is being used, the infant's mouth may have to be held shut to prevent air escaping during the procedure.

If there is difficulty achieving an effective breath, check the mouth for obstruction, reposition the airway (make sure the neck is not overextended) and make up to five attempts to achieve effective breaths. If still not successful then adopt the procedure for dealing with obstruction by a foreign body.

Chest compressions   The adult procedure is as follows:

- Kneel beside the patient, level with his/her chest and, using the hand nearest to the patient's feet, locate the lower rib edge by moving the index and middle finger to the mid-point where the ribs join the sternum.
- Place the middle finger over this point and the index finger next to it over the lower sternum.
- Place the other hand next to the index finger over the lower sternum, to locate the correct point for compressing the chest.
- Move the first-mentioned hand and place the heel of the hand on top of the hand over the lower sternum. Extend and lock the fingers, to keep pressure off the ribs.
- Keep the arms straight and press downwards to compress the chest by 4–5 cm[4].
- Release the pressure and then repeat the process of compressions at a rate of about 100/minute.
- Position the airway and give two effective breaths.
- Resume the compressions and rescue breaths in the ratio of 15:2.

The procedure for a child is as follows:

- Place the heel of one hand over the lower half of the patient's sternum and lift the fingers off his/her chest.
- Keep your arm straight and compress the sternum to about 1/3 to 1/2 the depth of the chest.
- Release the pressure and continue compressions at the rate of about 100/minute.
- After five compressions position the airway and give one effective breath.
- Resume the compressions and rescue breaths in the ratio of 5:1.

It may be necessary to use the two-hand procedure to obtain adequate compressions for a child aged over eight years. A ratio of 15 compressions to 2 rescue breaths should be used.

The procedure for an infant is as follows:

- Place two fingers over the sternum, one finger's width below the nipple line, and depress the sternum to about 1/3 to 1/2 the depth of the infant's chest.
- Release the pressure and continue the process at a rate of 100/minute.
- After five compressions position the airway and give one effective breath.
- Resume the compressions and rescue breaths in the ratio of 5:1.

Where two or more professionals are present, one may carry out the rescue breathing while the other performs the chest compressions using both thumbs over the lower half of the sternum with the hands encircling the infant's chest.

Basic Life Support   The *Resuscitation Guidelines* give advice about when to go for help. In an emergency in the practice there would usually be someone else present, who would be asked to ring for an ambulance as soon as it is realised a patient is not breathing. Details of the patient's age, reason for collapse, if known, and the practice address must be given. The aim of basic life support is to maintain the circulation of oxygenated blood until advanced life support measures can be taken. Do not stop the resuscitation procedure to check for a pulse (unless the patient moves). Keep going until the ambulance arrives or until the rescuer is exhausted.

Asphyxia

Blockage of the airway, so that the brain is starved of oxygen, can occur in ways ranging from inhalation of a foreign body, to crush injuries in an accident. Oxygen and suction could be needed. An asphyxiated patient loses consciousness quickly and the face and extremities become cyanosed. Death will follow if prompt action is not taken. The history might make the diagnosis obvious, e.g. the mother sees a child sucking something and the child then chokes and goes blue. However, in other situations such as an unconscious patient, the cause may not be known. A patient who develops respiratory distress while eating could have a foreign body obstruction but be mistakenly thought to be having a heart attack. An ambulance should be called as soon as the severity of the situation has been assessed and emergency help deemed necessary. The *Resuscitation Guidelines* include the procedures for dealing with choking in adults and children.

Choking

A patient who is breathing and coughing should be encouraged to clear the obstruction him/herself. If the obstruction cannot be cleared and the patient is becoming exhausted, intervention may be needed. The aim should be to artificially increase the pressure within the chest cavity to force the expulsion of the obstruction.

Infants (up to 1 year of age)   The procedure is as follows:

- If possible, position the baby in the prone position with the head lower than the chest, to make use of gravity to dislodge the obstruction and make sure it is does not pass further down the airway. Smaller infants can be held head-down along the rescuer's forearm. The jaw must be supported correctly to maintain the airway in the open position.

- Tap sharply between the baby's shoulder blades up to five times with appropriate force, to try to dislodge the foreign body.
- If the obstruction is not dislodged turn the infant into the supine position and perform up to five chest thrusts, using two fingers to compress the sternum at a point one finger's breadth below the nipple line. Chest thrusts should be performed more sharply and slowly (three second intervals) than those used for cardiac resuscitation. The intention in this instance is to force air out of the lungs in order to expel the foreign body.
- Check the mouth and carefully remove the foreign body if visible.
- Reposition the airway and check for breathing. If the infant is not breathing, attempt up to five rescue breaths to achieve two adequate ones.
- Repeat the procedure alternating five back blows with five chests thrusts, followed by rescue breaths, as the situation warrants. (Do not attempt abdominal thrusts on an infant because of the risk of rupturing abdominal organs.)

Children (over 1 year)   The procedure is as follows:

- Position in the prone position with the head lower than the chest and the jaw supported in the open airway position. It may be best for the rescuer to sit with the child across his/her lap.
- Give up to five back blows between the shoulder blades to try to dislodge the obstruction.
- If the obstruction has not been cleared give up to five chest thrusts. Place the child in the supine position with the head lower than the chest and position the airway. Place the heel of one hand over the sternum just below the nipple line. Keep the fingers away from the chest to avoid pressure over the ribs. Compress the sternum sharply and firmly at a rate of one every three seconds.
- Check the mouth and remove any visible foreign body carefully.
- Reposition the airway and check for breathing.
- If the child is not breathing try up to five rescue breaths to achieve two successful ones.
- If the obstruction has not been cleared repeat the entire procedure but alternate five abdominal thrusts with the five chest thrusts in each cycle. If the child is conscious and able to stand, the rescuer should get behind him/her and press sharply inwards and upwards with one hand below the xiphisternum. The necessity to kneel down to do this and the degree of pressure exerted will depend on the size of the child. If the child is unconscious, perform abdominal thrusts when recumbent. The intention of the procedure is to create pressure under the diaphragm to force air out of the lungs and expel the foreign body in the process.

Adults   The procedure is as follows:

- If the patient is conscious bend him/her forward with the head lower than the chest and support his/her chest with one hand.

- With the heel of the other hand, give up to five sharp blows midway between the patient's shoulder blades to try to dislodge the obstruction.
- If the obstruction is not cleared, perform up to five abdominal thrusts. Stand behind the patient, bend him/her forward and place the fist of one hand on the abdomen below his/her xiphisternum. Grasp the fist with the other hand and pull sharply upwards and inwards under the patient's ribcage.
- Repeat four more times if the first manoeuvres fail, and alternate with five back blows.
- If the patient loses consciousness at any time then remove any visible obstruction from the mouth, position the airway and check for breathing (the laryngeal muscles may relax after consciousness is lost).
- Attempt up to five rescue breaths to give two effective ones.
- If effective breaths are given then check for signs of a circulation and start chest compressions and/or rescue breaths as appropriate.
- If effective breaths are not achieved then give 15 chest compressions immediately to relieve the obstruction, without checking for signs of a circulation.
- Then check the mouth, remove any obstruction and attempt further rescue breaths.
- Continue giving 15 compressions and attempts at rescue breaths as appropriate.

Management of other emergency situations

Anaphylaxis

Anaphylactic shock is a life-threatening condition caused by an acute allergic reaction. The allergen causes histamine and other powerful substances to be released from mast cells which then cause: urticaria, peripheral vasodilatation and oedema, laryngeal stridor, bronchospasm and tachycardia. The patient may have a characteristic sense of impending death. The blood pressure falls and vital organs are starved of oxygen.

The action to be taken in such an event must be established in advance, with a protocol and emergency drugs always available. Request an emergency ambulance once anaphylaxis has been diagnosed, but initiate the treatment immediately. In March 2001 the Resuscitation Council UK published revised guidelines for community staff on the emergency treatment of anaphylaxis, which brought into line the recommendations of the *BNF*, the Green Book and the Resuscitation Council (UK)[5]. Every practice should have a copy of these guidelines and the treatment algorithms.

Action	Rationale
Lie the patient flat with legs raised if this does not exacerbate respiratory distress	To aid the venous return, although a dyspnoeic patient may not be able to lie down
Administer IM epinephrine (adrenaline) in the appropriate dose (see below)	To constrict peripheral blood vessels to raise the BP, and relieve bronchospasm
Check ABC	To assess the response to treatment
Begin CPR if needed	To maintain blood and O_2 to vital organs
Repeat epinephrine after five minutes	If there is no improvement
Transfer the patient to hospital	Delayed reactions may still occur

Doses of epinephrine (adrenaline) 1:1000 solution These should be given as follows:

- Less than 6 months   50 micrograms IM (0.05 ml)
- 6 months–6 years   120 micrograms IM (0.12 ml)
- 6 years–12 years   250 micrograms IM (0.25 ml)
- Over 12 years + adults 500 micrograms IM (0.5 ml).

Consult the guidelines for the acceptable dosage of Epipens (adrenaline solution in a disposable self-injection device).

If anaphylaxis occurs after an injection, save the syringe and vial if possible, in case they are needed for examination. A yellow card reporting an adverse drug reaction must be sent by the GP to the Committee on Safety of Medicines.

Fainting (vasovagal syncope)

Probably the commonest cause of collapse in the treatment room is a faint. Most patients get some warning of this. They become very pale and sweaty and feel nauseated; they may become confused, shaky or lose consciousness. The pulse will be slow. If a patient who feels faint lies flat or sits with the head lowered between the knees, this will often prevent the faint from occurring. (Note: a very pregnant woman should lie on her side because the enlarged uterus can compound the problem by slowing the venous return.) A patient who has collapsed from a simple faint will quickly recover when horizontal and this can be a useful diagnostic pointer to the cause of the collapse.

Myocardial infarction

Patients with severe angina or a frank myocardial infarct will sometimes arrive in surgery unaware how ill they are. The classical symptoms are severe, crushing, central chest pain with or without radiation to the jaw and left arm.

The patient may feel very unwell and look pale and sweaty. However, these gross symptoms are not always present and a patient may collapse without warning. In either case, assess the situation and call for an ambulance if no doctor is on the premises. If the patient is conscious obtain as much information as possible to help make the diagnosis. Sit the patient in the most comfortable position to assist his/her breathing; and if the patient carries glyceryl trinitrate or similar medication administer a dose to increase the cardiac perfusion[6]. If MI is suspected give the patient one aspirin (300 mg) to chew, for its anti-thrombotic effect (if no contraindications)[7]. Check the pulse and blood pressure to monitor progress and identify a deteriorating condition. Record an ECG and insert an IV cannula if possible.

In the event of cardiac arrest, follow the procedure set out above (under Collapse). Prompt defibrillation during the early stage of myocardial infarction is most likely to lead to a successful outcome. All practices are recommended to have an automated external defibrillator, with the staff trained to use it[8].

When no doctor is immediately available and an emergency call is received for a patient who has collapsed at home with symptoms suggestive of a myocardial infarction, then call an ambulance immediately.

Transient ischaemic attack

Atherosclerosis may affect the whole arterial tree in some older patients. From time to time this may result in the normal physiological mechanisms for maintaining the blood flow to be slightly delayed; the cerebral circulation is particularly sensitive in this situation. A sudden change in posture, turning the head quickly or other quick movement may cause the patient to be transiently giddy or even faint, but recovery is almost instantaneous. Patients can usually be reassured and advised to try and change position more slowly. The blood pressure should be recorded and referral made to the GP. Prophylactic aspirin could be needed to prevent more serious cerebral events.

Collections of platelets over atheromatous plaques can break off, lodge as emboli in the cerebral circulation and cause mild stroke symptoms. Recovery can take about 24 hours as the emboli disperse, but the process is likely to be frightening for the patient and carers. A medical examination will be necessary.

Cerebrovascular episode (stroke, CVA)

Another of the targets in *Saving Lives: Our Healthier Nation* is the reduction of the death rate from stroke in people aged under 75 by at least two fifths by 2010[9]. This may be achieved by identifying people at risk, controlling hypertension, giving prophylactic aspirin and promoting healthier lifestyles. However, the unfortunate patients who do suffer a stroke will need appropriate care.

A cerebral thrombosis, embolus or haemorrhage can cause a cerebral cata-strophe resulting in unconsciousness, hemiparesis or hemiplegia. The action to take if it occurs in the surgery is that for a collapsed patient. If it occurs at home, the relatives should be advised to make the patient as comfortable as possible wherever he/she has fallen, to maintain a clear airway, and to turn the patient into the recovery position if unconscious and breathing. The decision about admission to hospital should be made after all the circumstances have been considered, but it may be possible to wait until a doctor has seen the patient.

Convulsions

Epileptic seizures

A generalised seizure can be frightening both for the patient and any onlookers. A practice nurse's role can involve more than simply helping a patient who has a seizure in the surgery. Some practice nurses are using their expertise to give longer-term support to patients with epilepsy and their families. In the event of a tonic-clonic seizure in the surgery the principles are straightforward:

Action	Rationale
Give the patient as much room as possible and try to ease the fall	To prevent injury from hitting furniture or sharp corners
Protect the patient's head with a pillow if possible	To prevent unnecessary trauma
Do not attempt to wedge anything in the patient's mouth	More damage is likely to be caused and there is a danger of being bitten
Note the time and sequence of events	To aid the diagnosis – especially if a first fit
Move the patient into the recovery position once the seizure is over	To protect the airway until consciousness is regained

Once consciousness has been regained and the patient is talking coherently he/she can go home with a friend or relative, after verifying some details. The nurse must check whether the patient is taking medication regularly and has an adequate supply. A medical examination is usually needed for any patient after a seizure. Transfer to hospital should be arranged if repeated or uncontrolled seizures occur, or the patient does not regain consciousness after ten minutes.

Febrile convulsions

Babies and young children may develop convulsions in response to a febrile illness. A child will usually look hot, flushed and obviously feverish, with violent uncoordinated movements. Or he/she may be cyanosed from breath-holding, have twitching of the face and rolled up eyes.

Action	Rationale
Remove the child's clothing and check if the parents have administered paracetamol	To cool the skin by evaporation and to lower the body temperature with antipyretic treatment
Position the child on something soft	To prevent injury during convulsive movements
Explain to the parents what is happening	They are likely to be alarmed
Arrange for the child to be transferred to hospital if no doctor is immediately available	To identify and treat the cause of the fever

Tepid sponging has always been the traditional method for lowering the body temperature. It could be carried out while waiting for medical help if the procedure does not distress the child.

Head injury

A very young child and any patient who has been unconscious after a head injury, must be examined by a doctor. However, a practice nurse may sometimes see an active, alert child whose mother wants reassurance after the child sustained a fall or blow to the head. The assessment of a head injury should:

- Establish the circumstances of the injury
- Ensure there was no loss of consciousness, or any other injuries
- Ask if the patient remembers what happened
- Ask if the patient has felt dizzy or nauseated, or has vomited
- Check that vision is normal
- Check for sign of cerebral compression (e.g. fixed, dilated pupil)
- Check for CSF leaking from the nose or ears.

Cerebral compression may occur at the time of injury as a result of trauma to the brain, but can also develop some time after a head injury if a subdural haematoma forms[10]. Clear instructions about what signs to look for must be given before a patient goes home. Mild headaches, dizziness or irritability are not unusual after a head injury. If the symptoms persist or get worse; or if severe vomiting, limb weakness, severe drowsiness, increasing irritability, convulsions or photophobia develop, the patient must go to the hospital accident and emergency department for assessment.

Hypoglycaemia

Patients with diabetes treated with insulin are always at risk of having a hypoglycaemic attack, and should be aware of this. Part of their education about diabetes is to explain the risks of hypoglycaemia and each patient and his/her family should know the early signs so that action can be taken before unconsciousness supervenes.

The first sign of an impending hypoglycaemic attack is usually a feeling of faintness and hunger. This quickly passes on to confusion, aggressive behaviour and finally coma. The patient is pale, sweating and restless. Occasionally convulsions can occur, which can be mistaken for an epileptic seizure. The hypoglycaemic coma is a true emergency because the longer the patient is unconscious, the greater the risk of permanent brain damage from the low blood sugar. Thus the aim of immediate treatment is to raise the blood sugar to a normal level using the following procedure:

- If the patient is conscious give approximately 10 g of easily digested carbohydrate, e.g. two teaspoons of sugar or glucose, three glucose tablets, or 100 ml Lucozade.
- Follow up with 10–20 g of complex carbohydrate once the patient has recovered, e.g. 1–2 digestive biscuits or 150–300 ml of milk. Alternatively the patient should be advised to have a snack or meal if it is due.
- Hypostop (Glucose gel 10 g/23 g oral ampoule) dextrose gel in a tube can be squeezed inside the patient's cheek, to be absorbed through the buccal mucosa.
- Intramuscular glucagon can be given to an unconscious patient, followed by 30 g carbohydrate once consciousness is regained.
- The GP may need to give intravenous dextrose if all else fails.

The patient should be reviewed after a hypoglycaemic incident, to try and identify the cause and see if adjustments are needed to the treatment, diet, or lifestyle. Patients who are prone to hypoglycaemia should wear or carry something to identify them as having diabetes, e.g. Medic Alert bracelets or medallions.

Respiratory problems

Hyperventilation

Over-breathing can be associated with anxiety or emotional distress. Rapid, deep breathing can cause faintness, trembling and carpo-pedal spasm as carbon dioxide is breathed out and the acid/base balance is disturbed. The symptoms can cause further anxiety and so exacerbate the problem. A firm but quiet manner should be adopted. Take the patient to a quiet room, to help him/her to calm down. Try to establish what has happened. Other causes of respiratory distress need to be ruled out. Re-breathing carbon dioxide in expired air will restore the P_{CO_2} to its correct level, so if necessary, the patient can be encouraged to breathe in and out of a bag. Once the patient has recovered, help can be offered to try and deal with the underlying problems.

Acute asthma

There are always likely to be some patients who require emergency treatment for an acute attack of asthma, despite the general improvements in asthma management. Practice nurses should have a protocol to follow in the event of an emergency when a doctor is not present. The following should be assessed:

- Age of the patient and previous history – is the patient known to have asthma?
- Details of the present episode – duration, and any treatment already taken? Are there any known trigger factors?
- Degree of respiratory distress – is the patient able to talk?
- Are accessory muscles being used to breathe?
- Is the patient cyanosed?
- Peak expiratory flow rate (in comparison with the predicted level) if able to use a PEFR meter (see Chapter 6).
- Check pulse and respiration rates – there may be tachycardia and rapid respiration.
- Listen to the chest with a stethoscope for wheeze (if have been taught to do so).

Action	Rationale
Call for medical help (or an ambulance if the patient's condition warrants it)	This could be a medical emergency
Nebulise with salbutamol (2.5 mg for children, 5 mg for adults) or administer salbutamol via a spacer)	For the relief of bronchospasm
Monitor the patient's pulse and appearance while using the treatment	To detect any changes or deterioration in the patient's condition
Recheck the PEFR, pulse, respiration and chest sounds after 15 minutes	To determine the effectiveness of the treatment

Once the bronchospasm has been relieved, the patient should see a doctor or be treated by an experienced asthma nurse. Steroids are usually needed to deal with the inflammation of the airways. Admission to hospital may be necessary, but in any event, the patient will need a follow-up appointment. (See Chapter 16 under asthma management.)

Single-patient use nebuliser attachments must be replaced after use; reusable parts must be cleaned and autoclaved according to the instructions of the manufacturer.

Beta-agonist treatment used with a spacer has been shown to be at least as effective as nebulisers for adults, and to have some advantages compared to nebulisers for children with acute asthma[11].

Haemorrhage

Most cuts and minor haemorrhages will soon stop if simple pressure is applied to the site of bleeding. Gloves must be worn when dealing with any bleeding because of the risk of blood-borne infections.

Arterial bleeding

The bleeding will be profuse if an injury has severed an artery. The blood will be bright red and pumping out of the wound. Local pressure is the first act, followed by elevation of the limb, where relevant. Occasionally pressure will have to be exerted over the artery supplying the wound area. For example, in the groin, compress the femoral artery against the symphysis pubis, or in the upper arm, compress the brachial artery against the humerus. In an open wound an artery can sometimes be seen to be bleeding. If this is the case, then the direct application of an artery forceps to the cut end is the most effective way to control the bleeding. If the blood volume is reduced significantly, the patient will become shocked, with a weak rapid pulse and fall in blood pressure. Urgent transfer to hospital will be needed. Meanwhile lay the patient down and elevate his/her legs, if possible, to aid the venous return. Make sure there is no tight clothing and keep the patient warm but not overheated. Do not give anything to drink because an anaesthetic may be necessary, or vomiting may obstruct the airway if consciousness is lost.

Varicose veins

Occasionally a patient with varicose veins will knock his/her leg and puncture a vein. The bleeding is impressive but, being venous the blood is darker, slower flowing and not pumping out. The wound itself may be almost invisible but still bleed copiously. The treatment is simple: lay the patient down, put a pad on the wound, elevate the leg and wait for the bleeding to stop. After the patient has been lying down for half an hour with the leg elevated, a firm pad and bandage can be applied, and the patient may go home if medically fit. An appointment should be made for review of the wound. The management of varicose veins and the use of support stockings can then be discussed.

Haematemesis

Haematemesis is unlikely to occur in the surgery, but occasionally a call may be received. Most episodes of vomiting blood are significant but not desperately urgent; unless a large and obvious quantity of blood has been lost, when the patient will rapidly become shocked. This call requires urgent hospital admission, but more minor cases can be reassured and rested until a doctor can assess them.

Swallowed blood from the posterior nasal space is often mistaken for haematemesis and this cause should be considered. Taking an accurate history usually clarifies the issue.

Melaena

Bleeding within the bowel can often be overlooked in a patient who collapses from no apparent cause. A more common presentation is an unexplained iron-deficiency anaemia. Non-steroidal anti-inflammatory drugs are a common cause of gastrointestinal bleeding, especially in the elderly. Stool samples for occult blood may be requested if bleeding is suspected. The traditional black, tarry stool of the severe melaena makes recognition of the problem easy for the doctor or nurse. Patients with frank melaena require further investigations in hospital. A doctor should examine all patients with unexplained bleeding. Bright blood may come from haemorrhoids, but the possibility of a malignancy should always be considered.

Epistaxis

Nosebleeds are very common, particularly in children. A practice nurse may have to give advice over the telephone or to deal with the situation in the surgery. A calm manner will help to reassure the patient.

- Seat the patient with his/her head forward to prevent blood from running down the back of the throat.
- Instruct the patient to pinch the fleshy part of the nose between his/her finger and thumb for a timed ten minutes and to breathe through the mouth. This action should compress the bleeding point long enough to allow clotting to take place. It is not possible to guess the time accurately enough – a clock or watch must be used.

This action will stop a very high proportion of nosebleeds in children and some adults. A clot which has formed in the nostril should be left alone and not blown out as this will restart the bleeding. Recurrent nosebleeds in children are often due to a dilated single capillary in the lower part of the nasal septum. Excessive dryness of the mucosa and trauma, including nose-picking, can lead to bleeding. The treatment may be by cautery with silver nitrate or the use of antiseptic creams[12].

In adults the bleeding sometimes occurs from higher up the nose and may be precipitated by the rupture of a small arteriosclerotic capillary. Hypertension should be ruled out as a cause of a nosebleed. It is always worth recording the blood pressure and pulse. This can become useful information if the bleeding becomes profuse. Patients with bleeding disorders, who develop epistaxis, need urgent medical treatment. If the simple pressure technique does not stop the bleeding, then the nose may need to be packed; either by a doctor in the surgery or in an ENT department. Occasionally patients need hospital admission if the bleeding will not stop.

Poisoning

Young children will put anything in their mouths. An anxious parent may rush to the surgery for help when an accident occurs. If a patient is unconscious or known to have ingested a really hazardous substance, then call for an emergency ambulance immediately. Otherwise try to calm the situation and collect as much information as possible including what was taken how much, and when.

- <u>Do not</u> try to induce vomiting – caustic substances can cause further damage to the oesophagus, and volatile substances may affect the lungs.
- Consult the TOXBASE database for information about the risks and management of the poisoning incident. The practice should be registered with the site (see *BNF*[13]).
- If there is no GP available, consult the local accident and emergency department for advice about common poisons or suspected drug overdose.
- Consult the regional poisons information centre if more specialised advice is needed.
- Save any vomit in case it is needed for analysis.

This action would apply equally to adults who have been poisoned, either accidentally or through drug overdose. The abuse of alcohol, drugs and solvents can cause a patient to collapse and should be considered as a possibility.

Pain

Individuals have different tolerance levels for pain but a patient who attends the surgery with symptoms of pain will require a careful assessment. The nerve pathways and factors which influence the perception of pain are complex. The method of pain relief will vary with its cause, and if a nurse is required to assess a patient's pain, the following points should be considered:

- Type of pain – constant or intermittent, throbbing, burning, stabbing.
- Onset and duration – how long has the patient been in pain?
- Does anything help – position, analgesics, antacids?
- Intensity of pain, on a scale of 1–10, with 1 as very mild, to 10 as the worst pain imaginable.
- Localisation – can the patient show where the pain is?
- Appearance – posture, tension of facial muscles.
- Local signs – swelling, bruising, inflammation, deformity of joints.

Mild pain may be amenable to self-medication with simple analgesics, such as paracetamol. Localised pain from a wound may be relieved once it is dressed; or from an abscess once it is drained. Referral to the doctor will be necessary for patients with more severe pain. Alternative therapies may be effective in managing chronic pain. Some practice nurses are developing expertise in reflexology, therapeutic massage or acupuncture.

Trauma and minor injuries

Many of the conditions seen by a nurse in general practice will be minor injuries but they are included in this chapter because a few will have the potential to be life-threatening or to cause permanent disability. A practice nurse who treats a patient following an injury has a duty to ensure that the patient receives the most appropriate advice and treatment. A doctor should be consulted if there is any doubt about the diagnosis or management. Whenever a patient sustains a tetanus-prone wound, the patient's anti-tetanus immunisation must be checked and a booster or primary course given if needed (see Chapter 10 under immunisation).

Abrasions

The superficial skin loss caused by friction can be very painful because the sensory nerve endings in the skin are exposed. Thorough cleaning of the wound with water or saline is needed because residual grit can discolour the skin after healing. It may be possible to remove some particles from the wound by using fine splinter forceps. Wounds with deeply embedded dirt, especially on the face, may need to be cleaned under anaesthetic to prevent tattooing of the skin[14].

A suitable non-adherent or occlusive dressing will be needed to protect the wound and promote epithelialisation (see Chapter 5 under dressings).

Lacerations

The arrest of haemorrhage is discussed above. Most simple lacerations can be sutured in the treatment room. In general, all wounds which are gaping, especially on the scalp, fingers and over joint surfaces, will need suturing[15]. Some nurses have been taught to suture, and may be authorised to do so in the surgery. Reimbursement for sutures and local anaesthetics can be claimed on prescription as personally administered items. The use of sterile adhesive strips has reduced the number of injuries which need suturing. Tissue adhesive is also ideal for many wounds, especially in children, and the glue is now available on prescription. If a patient has sustained a tetanus-prone wound, his/her anti-tetanus status should be checked and immunisation offered as appropriate.

Burns and scalds

The immediate first aid treatment for a burn or scald is to put the affected area into cold water. Cold immersion considerably reduces the amount of tissue damage produced by heat[16]. If redness only has occurred and the area is small then probably no treatment except analgesia will be needed. An emollient cream will prevent itching as the skin heals. Sunburn is commonly seen in the treatment room as a first or even second degree burn. Soothing creams or aftersun lotion may be sufficient if blistering has not occurred. A patient with severe sunburn should see a doctor.

The possibility of non-accidental injury should always be borne in mind if the history is not consistent with the injury, there has been a delay of more than 12 hours in seeking treatment, or there are any other grounds for suspicion.

When blistering occurs after a burn or scald, the blisters should be left intact if possible, but they may have to be punctured with a sterile needle and the serum expressed. A suitable dressing should be applied if it is needed. Low-adherent dressings and film dressings are suitable for burns with little exudate. Patients who have extensive or deep burns should be treated in hospital to prevent or minimise scarring or contractures.

Soft tissue injuries

More soft tissue injuries are likely to be seen as patients are encouraged to take more exercise[17]. They need to be given advice about sensible exercise for their age and general condition and to understand the importance of doing warm-up exercises. Strains and sprains cause swelling, bruising and pain in the affected tissues. The history will often make the situation clear. Sometimes a fracture may also be suspected and must be treated accordingly. The initial treatment for a soft tissue injury includes:

- Rest – to avoid further damage to the tissues.
- Ice – to constrict peripheral blood vessels to reduce bruising and oedema, e.g. a small pack of frozen peas or purpose-made cold pack applied for five to ten minutes three to four times a day.
- Compression – to reduce the swelling and provide support, e.g. crepe bandage or double tubular elastic bandage (Tubigrip®).
- Elevation – to drain oedema by gravity and relieve pain[18].

Patients may be referred to a physiotherapist for treatment.

Fractures

Patients who have an obvious fracture will usually be transported directly to an accident and emergency department. However, minor fractures may be presented in the treatment room, often associated with other trauma such as bruises, sprains or lacerations. Particular care is needed with hand injuries because lasting deformities could result if not treated adequately. It is important to check that the tendon has not been affected in a finger injury. If there is any tenderness in the snuffbox area (the hollow between the base of the thumb and index finger) the injury must be treated as a scaphoid fracture until proved otherwise. These fractures cannot always be seen radiographically and a missed fracture could cause a long-term problem to the hand.

Stings and bites

Human and animal bites can often become infected, so the patient may need antibiotics as well as treatment for the wound. Tetanus immunity should be checked, and in the case of human bites, the patient may also require immunisation against hepatitis B. A blood test may be taken from a patient who has had a human bite, to test for blood-borne viruses. A second test will be needed three months later. The possibility of rabies should be considered if an animal bite occurred abroad.

Insect bites

Insect bites are usually easy to diagnose as the lesions are single, or in a cluster, and very irritating. Some bites cause a blister to form in the centre of the area bitten. Uncomplicated bites can be treated with 1% hydrocortisone cream plus antihistamine tablets, if the irritation is intense. The risk of malaria should be considered if a patient returns from a tropical area with mosquito bites. Patients need to understand the reason for completing any malaria prophylaxis regime.

Wasp and bee stings

Insect stings usually cause pain in the lesion but require little treatment in the majority of cases. A bee may leave the sting behind and this will need to be removed. Grasp the sting horizontally with forceps, below the poison sac, as close to the skin as possible and lift the sting out without squeezing the sac. Topical applications of a sting relief product can provide reassurance and may ease the discomfort. Hydrocortisone cream 1% will help to reduce the local inflammation, and antihistamine tablets may be needed if the reaction is more severe. If a patient is stung in the mouth, ice should be given to suck to reduce the swelling. Transfer to hospital should be arranged if there is any risk of oedema obstructing the airway. In rare cases of severe allergy, an anaphylactic reaction can occur. Patients to whom this has happened should carry adrenaline injections with them everywhere throughout the summer months, and know what to do in an emergency.

Ticks

These little insects are found in long grass and woodlands. They feed off animals and can attach themselves to exposed human skin. They bury their head in the skin and grow in size as they suck blood. It is important to remove the insect without leaving the head-part still buried. Plaster remover or spirit applied to the tick should make it withdraw backwards. It can then be removed with forceps, by using sideways movements to release the head from the skin. Alternatively, cover the tick with white soft paraffin and a film dressing. The tick will withdraw from the skin from lack of oxygen. The site should be cleaned well after the removal of the tick. Ticks can cause Lyme disease and other diseases, so the patient should be told to see the doctor and to mention the removal of the tick if a rash develops at the site of the tick-bite or he/she becomes unwell within the next fortnight.

Eye problems

The eye may be affected by an infection, foreign body, direct force or penetrating injury. A careful examination is needed and referral for medical treatment, in all but the most straightforward cases.

Conjunctivitis

This is a common condition with a variety of causes. The signs are:

- Painful or gritty red eyes with inflammation across the conjunctiva making the eye look pink; one or both eyes may be affected
- Discharge which may be purulent or just excessive tears
- The vision is unaffected.

The most common causes of conjunctivitis are infective or allergic. Very young babies can get conjunctivitis or a discharge from the eye because the tear duct system is not fully developed until the baby is about six months old. A few blocked tear ducts eventually require surgery. Advice may be needed on how to clean discharging eyes, using swabs soaked in cooled boiled water. Each swab to be used once and then discarded.

Bacterial eye infections cause a purulent discharge, which can be treated with antibiotic drops or ointment. Chloramphenicol is most commonly used. The condition is contagious and patients should be advised about hand-hygiene and the need to use separate towels and face flannels. Schools will usually exclude children until the infection has been treated[19]. If peri-orbital cellulitis occurs or the conjunctivitis is severe, the patient will need systemic antibiotics and to see a doctor urgently. Patients who wear contact lenses should be examined carefully to exclude trauma to the eye. The lenses should not be worn until the condition has completely resolved.

Allergic eye conditions can be caused either by hay fever or an allergy to make-up, in which case the product should not be used again. Antihistamine eye drops may be prescribed for the rapid relief of symptoms. Mast cell stabiliser drops such as sodium cromoglycate, are most useful for the prophylaxis of allergic eye symptoms. Oral antihistamines may also relieve allergic eye symptoms.

The important differential diagnosis for conjunctivitis is to exclude a foreign body from the surface of the eye. If a foreign body is suspected but not seen on examination then the eye should be stained with fluorescein drops to help identify a foreign body, corneal abrasion, or dendritic ulcer. The history of getting a piece of dust or similar material in the eye will give an important clue to a foreign body. Usually only one eye is affected and that will feel gritty or painful. The eye will be red and probably watering but in simple cases there will be no discharge.

Foreign bodies. Examine the eye carefully (see Chapter 5). Irrigation of the eye with saline may remove a foreign body. If it can be seen and is not embedded, then it may be possible to remove it with a moistened swab. A foreign body under the eyelid may be dislodged by drawing the upper lid over the lower lid so that the lower eyelashes sweep inside the lid. The upper lid can be everted by gently holding the stick of a cotton bud across the base of the tarsal plate of the eyelid while holding the eyelashes with the other hand and quickly drawing the eyelid outwards and upward over the cotton bud stick. No attempt should be made to remove a foreign body which is stuck or embedded. In such a situation, if no doctor is available, the patient should be referred to the ophthalmic casualty department for treatment.

Corneal abrasions occur if the cornea is scratched by a foreign body or a finger-nail. Fluorescein stains abrasions yellow/green where epithelial cells have been removed from the cornea. A blue-light pen-torch will illuminate a fluorescein-stained abrasion more easily.

Dendritic ulcers are caused by a herpes-like virus which can cause considerable damage to the eye if unrecognised. The symptoms are often identical to a foreign body – pain and a red eye. However, once stained, the ulcer appears as a tiny branching structure, more like the branches of a tree than the single line or mark of a corneal abrasion. Immediate medical referral is needed if an ulcer is seen.

Other causes of painful eyes. Of the many other causes of painful eyes which require referral, acute glaucoma is highly significant. In this condition the intra-ocular pressure rises, the cornea is often hazy, vision is poor and the patient is in pain. This is an emergency, as the eyesight can be seriously damaged. Chronic glaucoma is more common but does not usually present acutely. The onset is more insidious, possibly with headaches, but treatment is necessary to prevent loss of vision. (Patients who have a first-degree relative with glaucoma are entitled to free eye tests by an optician.) Herpes zoster (shingles) may present as pain in the eye or forehead before the typical eruption starts. Once the vesicles begin to develop the diagnosis is obvious; the patient should be referred for treatment urgently as soon as herpes zoster is suspected.

Foreign bodies

Nose

Children are remarkably adept at putting an assortment of items up their noses. The problem may become apparent because the child has obvious difficulty breathing through the nose, or a foul nasal discharge develops. If an object is small enough to go into the post-nasal cavity it can then fall down into the posterior pharynx and be inhaled into the airway. Thus, foreign bodies in the nose should be approached cautiously and the patient be referred to a doctor if the object cannot be removed easily with nasal forceps.

Ear

A similar assortment of items may be found in the external auditory meatus. It may be possible to remove a foreign body within view with a fine forceps, but if the removal is causing pain or bleeding, then the patient must be referred to the doctor. After removal of the object the drum and auditory canal should be examined carefully to exclude any trauma.

Vagina

A woman may ask the nurse to retrieve a lost tampon. A vaginal examination should be performed, and it may be possible to ease the tampon out if it can be felt easily. Often it is necessary to pass a vaginal speculum and use sponge-holding forceps to retrieve the object from the vaginal vault. Treatment may be necessary if the retained tampon has caused a bacterial vaginal infection.

Emergency midwifery

Although there would usually be time to summon help or transfer the patient to hospital, a nurse could be called upon to deliver a baby in the surgery in exceptional circumstances. For anyone without midwifery experience, the *First Aid Manual* has a good description and illustrations of what to do in an emergency[20]. This book is recommended for reference in all the situations which require first aid.

> ## Suggestions for reflection on practice
>
> - Review your emergency training and the surgery's emergency equipment:
>   - How well equipped do you feel to provide first aid or emergency treatment?
>   - What further training or resources do you require?
> - Audit the number of occasions you dealt with emergency situations over a chosen period of time.
>   - What was the outcome of your management?
>   - Could anything have been done differently?
> - Devise a survey to find out the circumstances under which a patient would choose to go either to an accident department or minor-injuries unit, or to the GP surgery.
>   - How will the results affect your practice?

Further reading

Resuscitation Council (UK) (2001) *Cardiopulmonary Resuscitation. Guidance for clinical practice and training in Primary Care. www.resus.org.uk/pages/cpatpc.htm* (accessed 10/8/01).

References

1. Department of Health (1999) *Saving Lives: Our Healthier Nation*. Department of Health, London.
2. Voluntary Aid Societies (1999) The ABC of life. In: *First Aid Manual*, revised 7th edn p. 41. Dorling Kindersley, London.
3. Resuscitation Council (UK) (2000) *Resuscitation Guidelines 2000*. Resuscitation Council UK, London.
4. Resuscitation Council (UK) (2001) *Depth of chest compression. www.resus.org.uk/pages/ccdepth.htm* (accessed 16/9/01).
5. Project Team of the Resuscitation Council (UK)(2001) *Update on the emergency medical treatment of anaphylactic reactions for first medical responders and for community nurses. www.resus.org.uk/pages/anaupdat.htm* (accessed 5/9/01).
6. Voluntary Aid Societies (1997) Heart attack. In: *First Aid Manual*, 7th edn, p. 83. Dorling Kindersley, London.
7. Mehta, S. (2001) Acute myocardial infarction. *Clinical Evidence*, **5**, 9–10. British Medical Journal Publishing Group, London.
8. Resuscitation Council (UK) (2001) *Cardiopulmonary resuscitiation guidance for clinical practice and training in primary care. www.resus.org.uk* (accessed 10/8/01).
9. Department of Health (1999) *Saving Lives: Our Healthier Nation*. Department of Health, London.

10. Walsh, M. & Kent, A. (2001) Head injury. In: *Accident and Emergency Nursing*, 4th edn, pp. 43–7.

11. Cates, J. & Rowe, B.H. (2001) Holding chambers versus nebulisers for beta-agonist treatment of acute asthma (Cochrane Review). In: *The Cochrane Library*, 3, Update Software, Oxford.

12. Burton, M. & Walton, R. (2001) Recurrent idiopathic epistastaxis (nosebleeds). *Clinical Evidence*, **5**, 274–6.

13. *BNF* (2001) Emergency treatment of poisoning. *British National Formulary*, **41**, 20–29. British Medical Association and Royal Pharmaceutical Society of Great Britain, London.

14. Small, V. (2000) Management of cuts, abrasions and laceration. *Nursing Standard*, **15** (5), 41–4.

15. Walsh, M. & Kent, A. (2001) Wound closure. In: *Accident and Emergency Nursing*, 4th edn. pp. 103–6.

16. Edwards, K. (1995) Burns. *Nursing Standard*, **10** (7), 27–9.

17. McHugh, M. (2000) Can exercise-induced muscle damage be avoided? *West Journal of Medicine*, **172** (4), 265–6.

18. NHS guidelines (1998) Sprains – general. *Prodigy Guideline, www.prodigy.nhs.uk/guidance/crs/Sprains-general* (accessed 19/9/01).

19. Mead, M. (2000) The illness conjunctivitis. *Practice Nurse*, **19** (5), 215–16.

20. Voluntary Aid Societies (1999) Emergency childbirth. In: *First Aid Manual*, revised 7th edn. pp. 197–202, Voluntary Aid Societies.

Useful addresses and web sites

Resuscitation Council UK
5th Floor Tavistock House North, Tavistock Square, London WC1H 9HR
Telephone: 020 7388 4678 Fax: 020 7383 0773
Web site: *www.resus.org.uk*

TOXBASE clinical toxicology database of the National Poisons Information Centre
Telephone: 0131 536 2298
Web site: *www.spib.axl.co.uk/*

National Poisons Information Service
Telephone: 0870 600 6266 (calls will be transferred to the nearest regional centre)

Chapter 8
Common Medical Conditions

Patients have several ways of getting help and advice with health problems, although the majority still tend to use their general practice.

NHS Direct is a 24-hour telephone helpline, manned by nurses, who will give advice at any time on any health issue. They use computerised protocols to assess the problems callers present and to give advice on the action needed. In some areas, calls to the GP out-of-hours service are answered by NHS Direct. The Government has expressed the intention of extending NHS Direct protocols to general practice in the future[1].

Nurse-run NHS walk-in and minor injury centres are intended to provide easy access to advice or treatment for patients with minor illnesses or injuries, to complement GP services[2]. Private health centres at main railway stations are used by commuters and people with limited time, who choose to pay for treatment rather than take time off work to visit their practice.

Nurse triage and the management of minor illnesses has become part of the role of many practice nurses. They assess the urgency of conditions when patients telephone or arrive at the surgery without an appointment, and give advice and treatment themselves or refer to the GP as appropriate. In this respect there is an overlap with the role of nurse practitioners.

A practice nurse may be consulted about a variety of common conditions. Some will be self-limiting illnesses, like colds and gastric upsets, for which advice can be offered on the management of symptoms. Other problems could necessitate referral to the doctor, who has the ultimate responsibility for medical treatment. Patients who attend frequently with seemingly minor problems may be looking for a chance to discuss a deeper worry. The doctor or nurse should provide the patient with a suitable opportunity to ventilate other concerns, especially if the consultation seems inappropriate for the symptoms presented.

Medication

The number of effective drugs available for purchase without a prescription changes periodically. Nurses may be asked for advice about suitable over-the-counter (OTC) medicines, so it is essential to enquire about any allergies, other medication being taken, possible pregnancy or other medical conditions before recommending proprietary products. As cost is a major factor for patients on low income, prescriptions may need to be issued for those who are exempt from prescription charges. Information leaflets should be available in the surgery about help with NHS prescription costs. Retail pharmacists will advise patients about a wide range of problems and treatments. A friendly pharmacist is also a valuable source of information for doctors and nurses. Primary care trust (PCT) pharmacists work closely with practices on a range of prescribing issues and are another resource for practice nurses.

Nurse prescribing

Nurse prescribing is currently only permitted for practice nurses with a district nursing or health visiting qualification who have passed the examination at the end of the nurse prescribing training[3]. Nurse prescribers are recorded with the UKCC. The products in the *Nurse Prescribers' Formulary* are severely limited. However, it will soon be possible for a larger number of nurses to prescribe within their sphere of expertise after suitable training, as either independent or dependent (supplementary) nurse prescribers[4]. The NHS plan expresses the intention that more than half of all nurses will be able to supply medicines by 2004.

The practice nurse's responsibility regarding prescriptions

The practice nurse has the following responsibilities in relation to prescriptions:

- To ensure that any prescription issued by the nurse is given to the correct patient
- To be able to answer knowledgeably, or refer to the appropriate person, any enquiries by patients about their medication
- To ensure that blank prescriptions are stored securely in the nurse's room
- To be familiar with the repeat prescribing system
- To have appropriate reference material available.

If patients are given advice by nurses on self-management they must be told to consult their GP if the condition worsens or does not resolve in the time expected. Verbal information is forgotten quickly, so important points can be reinforced with printed handouts or leaflets.

It is possible to give only a brief overview of some of the medical conditions with which practice nurses may be involved. So much depends on the circumstances in individual surgeries and the experience of the nurses concerned.

Upper respiratory tract infections

The majority of upper respiratory symptoms due to infection are caused by viruses. Antibiotics should only be required if secondary bacterial infection supervenes. Advice to patients includes:

- An explanation of the nature of viral infections.
- The value of analgesic/antipyretic compounds, such as aspirin or para-cetamol, in appropriate dosage (aspirin can cause Reye's syndrome and is not recommended for children under 12 years of age[5]).
- Suggestions about proprietary cough linctuses and decongestants. Remember to warn patients that antihistamines in some preparations can cause drowsiness. Pseudoephedrine is contraindicated for patients taking MAOI antidepressants and caution is needed if patients have diabetes, IHD, hypertension or hyperthyroidism.
- The need for regular drinks to prevent dehydration.
- Advice about the environment:
  - bedrest is not necessary unless the patient feels more comfortable there
  - central heating and crowded, smoky atmospheres can make symptoms worse
  - if apyrexial the only value in being away from work is to avoid passing the infection on to other people
- To consult the doctor if:
  - a fever persists
  - the sputum becomes discoloured (antibiotics may be required)
  - there is pain on inspiration (could indicate pleurisy)
  - earache or facial pain occur (could indicate infection of the ears or sinuses).

Smokers may be more receptive to offers of help to quit, while symptoms make them disinclined to smoke.

Catarrh

The term catarrh covers a multitude of disorders related to the sensation of congestion in the nasal airways, sinuses, or ears. Some patients suffer all the time (with perennial rhinitis or chronic sinusitis); others may have an acute problem related to hay fever or the common cold. The treatment will depend on the underlying cause. The patient's occupation should always be checked because there may be an acquired sensitivity to fumes, dust or chemicals at work. There could be health and safety implications[6].

Seasonal rhinitis (hay fever)

The symptoms of hay fever: itchy, watering eyes, sneezing, blocked or running nose, and sometimes wheezing chest, are caused by an allergic reaction to pollen or mould spores. Atopic individuals have an inherited tendency to develop hay fever, asthma and eczema. Patients known to suffer from seasonal rhinitis are advised to start preventive therapy a fortnight before the hay fever season begins.

Treatments available The following treatments may be used (some treatments are not suitable for children):

- Antihistamines are used to relieve the symptoms. Cetirizine, fexofenadine, loratadine, are newer antihistamines which are said to not cause drowsiness, whereas with products like chlorpheniramine and promethazine, patients must be warned against driving or working with machinery.
- Mast cell stabilisers – sodium cromoglycate as eye drops, nasal spray, or inhaler as preventive measures.
- Steroids – beclomethasone, budesonide, fluticasone nasal sprays.
- Oral steroids may be prescribed in extreme cases but steroid injections are no longer recommended for hay fever[7].

Perennial rhinitis

Although the symptoms and treatment are similar to hay fever, people with perennial rhinitis suffer the symptoms all year. Instead of pollen they may be sensitive to allergens like house dust mites or animals. Advice can be given on ways of reducing the exposure to allergens. Nasal polyps should be ruled out as a cause of symptoms.

Ear conditions

A practice nurse should be able to visualise the external meatus of the ear and the tympanic membrane, and be familiar with the appearance of a normal ear. Children, in particular, are susceptible to middle ear infections following a cold and any child who complains of earache should be examined. If a practice nurse examines the ears and the drums are not absolutely normal then the child should be referred to the doctor for advice. Patients may be taught that anti-biotics are not helpful for viral ear infections[8]. However, it is important that they understand the importance of compliance (concordance) with any treatments prescribed.

Deafness

Blocked ears can be caused externally by excessive wax, debris from otitis externa, or foreign bodies; and internally by congestion of the middle ear. Ear irrigation might need to be performed (see Chapter 5). Decongestants such as pseudoephedrine may be recommended for congestion of the middle ear if the patient is otherwise well (see *BNF* for contraindications). In other circum-stances the patient should be referred to a doctor.

Headache

Patients with occasional headaches usually treat themselves with OTC analgesics. Most causes of headache are minor, but more serious disease has to be eliminated. Patients with headaches sometimes refer themselves to the practice nurse for a blood pressure check. A medical assessment should be arranged for a patient with recurrent or severe headaches, but once serious disease has been ruled out, the practice nurse can help the patient to deal with the symptoms and to devise avoidance strategies. Rebound headaches can occur as a result of larger amounts of analgesics, so some patients may inad-vertently be compounding the problem.

Migraine

There are several theories to explain the symptoms of migraine. The cause is still not fully understood. Episodic attacks of severe unilateral headache, nausea or vomiting, photophobia or other neurological disturbances, lasting for several hours or days are characteristic. Attacks can be preceded by a visual or sensory disturbance (aura) and migraine is classified as migraine with aura and migraine without aura. Sufferers have a family history of migraine in 70% of cases. A number of trigger factors – dietary, hormonal, emotional and environmental, are implicated and sometimes an accumulation of triggers will precipitate an attack. No diagnostic test exists, so a clear history of symptoms is needed. A migraine diary can aid diagnosis and help patients to identify possible trigger factors.

Treatment

There is no cure but drugs can sometimes be effective in preventing or relieving symptoms. Changes in lifestyle to avoid trigger factors, relaxation techniques and alternative therapies like acupuncture can be beneficial. Some nurses run migraine clinics with an holistic approach to the problem. Self-help groups also exist for sufferers.

Tension headaches

The sensation of a tight band around the head caused by tension in the neck muscles, can be eased by relaxation, stress reduction and massage. Analgesia may also be required.

Hangover

Headache following excessive alcohol intake is not uncommon. Practice nurses can give information to sufferers on sensible drinking (see Chapter 9) and advise on the prevention of a hangover by maintaining adequate hydration.

Insomnia

Clinicians are often requested by patients to prescribe something 'to help me sleep'. Many patients have a high expectation of a perfect night's sleep irrespective of age, other concomitant illness or their own personal needs. A great deal more is known now about sleep and the way various drugs affect it, and doctors are reluctant to prescribe drugs likely to cause addiction or habituation. Nurses may be able to help patients who are having difficulty in sleeping. Thorough assessment of the problem may present possible solutions:

- Daytime sleep. An elderly patient who has several short naps during the day will not sleep so well at night.
- Pain. People with severe pain sometimes request sleeping tablets, when adequate analgesia would be more effective.
- Mental distress. Counselling may be offered to patients with anxiety or other distress. People with severe depression could require treatment with anti-depressants.
- Nocturia merits investigation for urinary infection, diabetes, prostatism or the timing of diuretics.

It may also help to consider the sleeping environment – a warm milky drink, reading in bed and comfortable bedding all encourage the mind and body to wind down from the day's activities. Relaxation techniques can be taught. Quietness may take more innovation to achieve, especially if a partner snores. Ear plugs might provide relief, and ENT assessment of the snorer might be possible.

Gastrointestinal disorders

Diarrhoea and vomiting are common symptoms, particularly in children. While most of these episodes are relatively trivial and self-limiting, the risk of dehydration or the masking of more severe pathology, such as intestinal obstruction, always has to be borne in mind.

Causes

The causes of diarrhoea and vomiting are many. Age is an important consideration when trying to decide about likely cause and future management. Some of the common causes are:

Vomiting

- Viral, bacterial or toxic causes in all age groups
- Feeding problems in babies
- Middle ear or upper respiratory infection in children
- Pregnancy
- Ménière's disease or labyrinthitis in the middle-aged and the elderly, particularly if there have been previous episodes
- Migraine
- Gallstones
- Intestinal obstruction, particularly in babies and the elderly.

Diarrhoea

- Following vomiting, almost always infective and often viral
- On its own at any age, infection, occasionally from contaminated food (enquire about recent travel)
- Other bowel disorders such as ulcerative colitis; the length of history will usually give the clue to these conditions
- Spurious diarrhoea in the elderly, caused by faecal leakage around impacted faeces.

Management

- In simple uncomplicated cases where the patient is over one year of age and the history is only a matter of hours, then frequent small sips of fluid until bowel symptoms have subsided are all that is required (starvation is no longer recommended so the patient may eat a normal diet if desired).
- Advise the patients to contact the practice again if symptoms persist for more than 24 hours, if abdominal pain is persistent or severe, or blood is being passed.
- Children under a year old or any patients whose symptoms do not fit into the infective pattern should be referred to the doctor the same day.

Patients with diarrhoea who work as food handlers should be advised to stay away from work until 48 hours after the condition has resolved.

Dyspepsia

Probably more OTC remedies are bought for indigestion than for most other symptoms. Causes can include poor eating habits, pregnancy, hiatus hernia, smoking and high alcohol consumption. However, clinical diagnosis is difficult and patients with persistent symptoms will require medical investigations. The nurse may be the first person consulted, so any patient taking antacids regularly, having a lot of pain, or loss of weight, needs referral.

Constipation

Patients can become anxious if their bowels do not work regularly, as witnessed by the many tons of laxatives consumed annually. Normal bowel habits vary, so a diagnosis of constipation has to be related to the norm for each individual. The advice given will depend on the age group of the patient. However the possibility of intestinal obstruction should be considered when a patient has severe constipation. A thorough history must be taken before any advice or treatment is offered.

Babies often become constipated when their dietary intake is being changed, e.g. change from breast to bottle or milk to solids. An increase in the amount of fluid given (not just milk) may be all that is required. The health visitor will usually advise parents and refer to the GP if necessary. Young children may be slow to acquire normal toilet training habits. Health visitors will advise parents about toilet training. It is important not to focus too much attention on bowel function because a child can learn to exert power over parents by refusing to comply. Children can also be so absorbed in their daily activities that they forget to go to the toilet and so become constipated by suppressing the normal bowel reflexes. Fear of defaecation resulting from the experience of passing a painful stool or from an anal fissure can also lead to constipation.

Management of constipation in children

- Advise increased roughage in the diet (fruit purée, vegetables, high-fibre cereals and bread), and extra fluids
- Encourage regular, unhurried toileting and reward with praise
- Faecal softeners (e.g. docusate) and/or paediatric glycerine suppositories may be prescribed to relieve severe constipation; and anaesthetic gel to be applied around the anus to relieve the pain of defaecation.

Management of constipation in adults

Constipation in adults or the elderly can be acute or chronic. Acute constipation may be the result of activity restriction by illness or injury, dehydration, or drugs such as codeine. Long-term laxative use can cause chronic constipation. The bowel loses its muscle tone and reflexes, so a vicious circle is created whereby the bowel only functions when stimulated by purgatives. Poor diet and lack of exercise contribute to constipation in all age groups. Changes in bowel habits can be a sign of significant bowel disease, so constipation in a patient who has previously been regular; or alternating constipation and diarrhoea, requires medical investigation.

Management of acute constipation   This can be done in the following ways:

- Identify the cause, if possible, and ask for a medical examination if necessary
- Deal with the immediate problem, advise osmotic laxatives or glycerine suppositories in mild to moderate cases
- Advise on the prevention of a recurrence by the use of softening agents, increased fibre and fluids (if patients have to take drugs known to cause constipation, suitable laxatives will be needed as well).

Management of chronic constipation   This can be done in the following ways:

- Encourage gradual re-education of the bowel with changes in diet to increase fibre and fluids
- Change from stimulant laxatives to faecal softeners and bulking agents
- Encouraging patients to change the habits of a lifetime requires patience. (sudden increases in dietary fibre can cause distressing flatulence, which patients should be warned to expect and be reassured will settle once the body adjusts).

Worms

Harmless threadworms are the most common parasitic worms which inhabit the gut in Britain, especially in children. Roundworms and tapeworms are less common, but can cause anorexia, weight loss and abdominal distension. Travellers may occasionally return with other helminth infections. Threadworms, true to their name, look like small white threads. They inhabit the bowel and emerge at night to lay their eggs around the anus, causing intense irritation which can disturb sleep or cause bed-wetting.

Treatment should include all the family. Anthelmintic preparations can be bought over the counter or prescribed by the GP or a nurse prescriber. Piperazine can be given to children from one year of age (in a lower dose for children under six years old). Mebendazole is only suitable for children over two years old, but in the same dose for all age groups. The whole family should be treated at the same time but mebendazole is contraindicated for pregnant or lactating women (see *BNF*). The nurse has a role in teaching parents how to avoid reinfection. Information leaflets are available from local health promotion departments. Threadworms are spread by ingestion of the eggs from hand contact. Scratching the peri-anal skin will transfer eggs to the hands. Prevention therefore depends on hand hygiene, keeping fingernails short, and family members using their own face flannels and towels.

Urinary problems

Cystitis

The complaint of cystitis may mean anything from slight burning or frequency of micturition to severe pain, nausea and febrile illness. Cystitis is very common in women, and may or may not be associated with a proven urinary tract infection. Inflammation of the lower urinary tract is often associated with sexual intercourse. Changes in cell structure due to loss of oestrogen can also make post-menopausal women prone to cystitis. Organisms which colonise the bowel will cause infection if they gain entry to the urinary tract. Anatomical differences make this much less common in men; therefore, a medical assessment is needed for any man with a urinary tract infection. A pregnant woman with a urinary infection must also be seen by the doctor. Referral to the genitourinary clinic is advisable if cystitis is thought to be associated with a sexually transmitted disease.

Most urinary tract infections will be picked up with dip tests for nitrites and leucocytes and treatment with antibiotics may be initiated immediately in some instances. Blood may also be detected on urinalysis but is not necessarily diagnostic of infection, especially if a patient is menstruating. A midstream specimen of urine should be sent for microbiology, in accordance with the practice protocol. This might include all urinary tract infections or only those in specific patient groups: men, pregnant women, children and patients with haematuria or suspected kidney infections[10]. If an MSU is sent, the pathology form should specify any antibiotic prescribed so that sensitivity can be tested to that particular antibiotic.

Women who are prone to recurrent attacks of cystitis can be given information on ways to minimise problems:

- Wipe from front to back after using the toilet, to avoid bringing bowel organisms in contact with the urethra
- Avoid using scented soaps, bath products, talc and vaginal deodorants, which can irritate the skin
- Increase fluid intake to about four litres a day
- Empty the bladder regularly and completely
- Avoid restrictive clothing and tights, and wear cotton underwear in preference to nylon
- Use a lubricant if intercourse is affected by vaginal dryness
- If using a diaphragm ensure it is the correct size, to avoid pressure against the urethra (recurrent UTIs could necessitate a change of contraceptive method)
- Consult the doctor about hormone replacement for treatment of post-menopausal urinary symptoms
- If symptoms of cysitis begin, take an alkali – either a proprietary preparation from the chemist or a teaspoon of bicarbonate of soda in water hourly, for three hours, to alter the pH of the urine; as well as 500 ml of liquid every 20 minutes for the same length of time to dilute the urine and relieve irritation of the bladder mucosa.

Cranberry juice has been recommended or used for the treatment of urinary tract infections for some years. It is claimed that the tannins in cranberry juice prevent *Escherichia coli* from attaching themselves to the walls of the urinary tract[11].

However, a Cochrane Review has not found convincing evidence of the efficacy of cranberry juice[12]. More research is needed.

Cystitis in children

The situation with children is different. Undiagnosed infection, often due to an anatomical abnormality, can lead to low-grade pyelonephritis with no symptoms, which can ultimately cause renal scarring and possibly, eventual renal failure. Therefore it is vital to examine the urine of children and refer to the doctor if there is any likelihood of a urinary tract infection. Inefficient development of the valves at the ureto-bladder junction will allow reflux of urine up the ureters on micturition. If they can be kept free of infection, most children develop the use of these valves by eight to ten years of age. Prophylactic antibiotic treatment may be required with regular MSUs. Other causes of cystitis in children include vaginal infection or balanitis, foreign body, and worms. The possibility of sexual abuse also has to be borne in mind.

Vaginal discharge

Women have varying amounts of vaginal discharge present, either at certain times of the menstrual cycle or all the time. Infection can be caused by a variety of organisms, often sexually transmitted. Offensive discharge may result from a forgotten tampon or other foreign body. It is important to establish exactly what a woman is complaining about when she says she has a vaginal discharge. A high vaginal swab will usually be required to identify the cause of infection.

Candida albicans (thrush)

If the normal balance of commensal organisms is disturbed, an overgrowth of yeasts can result. Antibiotics, diabetes, pregnancy and the oral contraceptive are contributory factors. The characteristic white cheesy discharge of *Candida* infection is very irritant. Treatment is usually simple and consists of antifungal vaginal preparations such as clorimazole pessaries or cream. They may be bought over-the-counter or prescribed. Oral treatment, one capsule of fluconazole can be used for more intractable cases. The nurse can explain the condition to patients and advise on ways of preventing a recurrence:

- Avoid using scented soaps, talc etc. and avoid obsessive hygiene measures which remove the normal commensal flora
- Wear loose-fitting cotton underwear
- Wear stockings instead of tights
- Avoid tight-fitting jeans and trousers.

Bacterial vaginosis

Bacterial infections of the vagina can also cause an irritating discharge. Sometimes patients request a repeat of treatment for thrush, when the problem is in fact bacterial. A high vaginal swab should be sent when necessary. Most offending organisms can be treated with systemic metronidazole or topical preparations such as clindamycin cream.

Trichomonas vaginalis

Trichomoniasis is sexually transmitted by a flagellate organism and produces a frothy yellow discharge. Metronidazole taken orally for a week will provide effective treatment, but patients must be warned to totally avoid alcohol while taking it. Patients may also require persuasion to persevere with the treatment because it can cause such an unpleasant taste in the mouth and nausea.

Chlamydia

Another protozoa, *Chlamydia*, is a common cause of resistant vaginal discharge and pelvic inflammatory disease (see Chapter 12). Special swabs are required to identify the organism (see Chapter 6). Recognition and adequate treatment with antibiotics is essential because of the serious risk to future health and fertility.

General advice

Patients may have more than one sexually transmitted infection and referral to a genito-urinary clinic will sometimes be advisable. Unfortunately, the former stigma associated with these clinics may deter some patients. A practice nurse can help by explaining about the skilled diagnosis and treatment available at specialist centres, and by giving practical information about clinic times and location. Appropriate advice may also be given on hygiene, safer sex, contraception, and cervical screening (see Chapter 12, Sexual Health).

Infectious diseases

Many of the most common childhood illnesses can now be prevented by immunisation and are, therefore, seen only rarely. Patients may contact the practice nurse for information about the risk of contracting or spreading a disease, or for diagnosis of a skin rash. It will often be possible to identify the common conditions and give appropriate advice but this can be rendered extra difficult when patients want the rash to be identified by telephone.

Chicken pox (Varicella)

The characteristic lesion of chicken pox is a small blister-like spot with clear serous fluid in the centre. There may be many of these scattered over the trunk and face, showing various stages of development from an early red spot, through the vesicular stage, to crusting and the formation of a scab. The diagnosis will usually be obvious, especially as chicken pox tends to occur in minor outbreaks of cases. Apart from being febrile and irritable, a child is only very rarely at risk from complications. Treatment with calamine lotion may help to cool down the irritating spots. An antihistamine such as promethazine will reduce the itch and sedate the patient in more severe cases. It can help to put the child in a warm bath with sodium bicarbonate added to the water to reduce the irritation.

Chicken pox infection, in a non-immune woman, in the first two trimesters of pregnancy can cause severe congenital abnormalities in about 2% of cases. The critical period is between 13 and 20 weeks gestation[13]. Infection around the time of delivery poses a risk of overwhelming infection to the infant. This should be remembered if a pregnant woman seeks advice about chicken pox; a referral to the doctor may be necessary. If the mother has definitely had chicken pox there is no risk. Many cases in childhood are very mild. There may be no memory of the illness but a high proportion of adults do have immunity. If in doubt, an urgent blood test can be taken to check the antibody levels. A non-immune woman may be given varicella-zoster immunoglobulin.

Shingles (Herpes zoster)

Shingles occurs from the reactivation of varicella virus, dormant in the ganglion of a nerve since a previous episode of chicken pox, which then travels back down the nerve to affect the skin area (dermatome) served by that nerve. This is commonly around one side of the trunk but can occur on the head and seriously affect the eye. The old wives' tale about a patient dying if shingles meets in the middle arises from the rare cases of extremely debilitated people, who develop shingles affecting dermatomes on both sides of the body at the same time. Immunocompromised patients should be aware of the risk from shingles and know the importance of seeking medical treatment immediately.

It is possible for a person who has never had chicken pox to catch the disease from someone with shingles because the same virus is responsible for both, but shingles cannot be caught from chicken pox for the reason given above.

Shingles can cause severe pain requiring regular analgesia, which occasionally leads to post-herpetic neuralgia. Antiviral drugs can reduce the symptoms if taken within 72 hours of the onset of shingles and should be considered for patients over 60 years, in any patient with eye involvement, or shingles affecting the neck, limbs or perineum[14].

Measles

Measles has rarely been seen in recent years but it may become more common as a result of a reduction in the uptake of MMR vaccine; sadly some children in Ireland have already died as a result of measles[15]. The patient may be unwell and has usually been so for several days. He or she is catarrhal with a hard non-productive cough and a temperature of about 39°C. The eyes are often red and there is a blotchy, flat rash over the trunk, head and limbs. The rash often starts behind the ears and will slowly develop over the ensuing 24 hours. Koplik's spots look like tiny white grains of salt on the mucous membrane of the mouth and appear before the rash. They are thus a useful diagnostic pointer when measles is suspected. Laboratory diagnostic confirmation is usually required. The local consultant in communicable disease control will advise.

Mumps

Mumps is a viral infection spread by droplets which causes fever and painful swelling of the parotid glands. The incubation period can be up to three weeks. The resulting difficulty in eating and drinking can lead to dehydration in severe cases. Other organs can also be affected – the kidneys, pancreas, thyroid and the testes. Orchitis can result in sterility in a small proportion of the men who develop the disease. Meningitis is another complication of mumps, which is not usually life-threatening but requires careful monitoring. Treatment for mumps is symptomatic, with bed-rest while the fever is high and measures to reduce the fever and relieve pain. An adequate fluid intake is needed to avoid dehydration and constipation. The patient is infectious from about a week before the fever starts to the time the swelling subsides but close contact is usually needed for the disease to be transmitted.

German measles (rubella)

The rash of typical rubella is much more diffuse than measles and is often very striking on the face. The diagnosis should not be made if the posterior occipital chain of lymph glands cannot be palpated, as many virus infections produce a transient non-specific rash very similar to rubella. The rubella rash lasts for several days whereas the imitative virus infections seldom last more than 24 hours. No treatment is required and children only need to be kept out of contact with known expectant mothers. Children who did not receive MMR still need to be immunised even if they are thought to have had the clinical rubella infection, because a firm diagnosis is often difficult to make.

Slapped cheek syndrome (erythema infectiosum)

Also known as *fifth disease*, this is caused by a parvovirus, which mainly affects school-age children but can occur in adults. The infection, which is mainly spread by droplets, causes a red rash on the cheeks – hence the common name, and a mild flu-like illness. Itching can be troublesome and the rash may spread to other parts of the body. Adults may get swollen painful joints. The incubation period is 1–3 weeks. The disease is mild in children but can cause anaemia in a fetus or occasionally, miscarriage, if a pregnant woman passes the disease to her unborn child. In general, symptomatic treatment only is needed. Pregnant women should seek medical advice.

Hand, foot and mouth disease

This disease, not to be confused with foot and mouth disease of animals, is caused by a Coxsackie virus and mainly affects children. There may be fever and a sore throat followed by the development of small blisters in the mouth, hands and feet. Blisters can also occur on the buttocks. The disease is spread partly by droplets or from contact with virus in the blisters. Faecal/oral transmission is also possible because the virus is excreted in the faeces for some time after the infection. The incubation period is short 3–7 days. No treatment is needed but careful hygiene measures are required after toiletting young children with the disease.

Human parasites

Scabies (Sarcoptes scabiei)

Scabies is caused by the allergic reaction to a small arthropod which lays its eggs in burrows just below the surface of the skin. It can only be transmitted by direct skin contact with an affected person. It causes intense irritation and the classical burrow lesions can usually be found in the web of the fingers or the wrist. Although these are common sites, it must be assumed that the whole skin except the head will be affected. Crusted scabies often occurs in immunocompromised patients. It is extremely contagious and will affect the head and face as well.

Treatment choice depends on the patient's age and medical condition. All contacts should be treated at the same time to avoid reinfestation. Apply a scabicide cream or lotion (permethrin or malathion) from neck to toes, paying particular attention to the skin folds. Treatment should be reapplied to hands after hand washing. After 12 hours the whole body can be bathed. Treat all members of the household at the same time. Skin irritation will continue for several days after treatment. In heavily infected cases a further treatment will be needed after ten days.

Head lice (pediculosis capitis)

Head lice are common in all age groups but are found more often on children. They can occur in even the most scrupulously careful household and can engender concern out of all proportion to their effect. Head lice are usually first noticed as nits; the eggs which the female louse glues to individual hairs. Newly laid eggs will be close to the scalp, and those further away and white are hatched eggs which progress outwards as the hair grows. The louse itself is very small and difficult to see. It passes from one head to another by contact. If lice are discovered, the parent should inform the school, playgroup, or others in close contact.

   The patient and any family members who have been shown to have live lice, should be treated at the same time. A second application may be needed after ten days to kill any lice which hatched after the first treatment. Pregnant women must avoid using permethrin. Local policies exist for rotating treatments in an attempt to prevent resistance to insecticides. For this same reason regular preventive use of pediculosides must be discouraged. Education of the public to understand the problem and adopt simple measures, like weekly checks of children's hair with a special head lice comb for early detection is important. The value of bug-busting (regular wet-combing of hair treated with hair conditioner), has not been confirmed as an effective cure[16].

Crab lice (pediculosis pubis)

Body lice are usually found in the pubic hair and are more easily seen than head lice because they are larger (about the size of a pinhead). Infection occurs mainly with sexual contact. Treatment is by application of an appropriate lotion (phenothrin, malathion), left on for up to 12 hours and then washed off. All hairy areas of the body, including a beard, must be treated, according to the manufacturer's instructions, with an aqueous solution.

Other skin conditions

The appearance of the skin can affect the way a person is treated by society. Skin diseases are rarely life-threatening but they can devastate self-esteem. Up to 15% of consultations in general practice are related to skin conditions, so there is plenty of scope for nurses with specialist skills in dermatology to help patients to improve their quality of life[17].

Acne vulgaris

Puberty is never the easiest time to live through; but to develop acne, just when self-image becomes all important, must rank among the crueller tricks of Nature. Young patients with acne often need a lot of support and counselling. They should be encouraged to lead a normal social life, and to avoid using make-up to cover blemishes, as this will block sebaceous glands even more. It is a myth that a diet high in carbohydrate and fats will aggravate the situation, but the value of non-greasy foods and fresh fruit should be emphasised for general health reasons.

Preparations used in treating acne aim at reducing the grease in the skin, and the number of blocked sebaceous ducts (blackheads). Benzoyl peroxide removes the surface layer of skin to unblock the pores. Azelaic acid works in a similar fashion and also has antibacterial properties. All keratolytic products can make the skin dry and sore. A light moisturising cream may help if this occurs and treatment may also need to be stopped for a few days. Topical antibacterial products may be prescribed in some instances for inflammatory acne but antibacterial resistance can occur (see *BNF*).

In more severe acne with persistent pustules and spots on the face and shoulders the doctor may prescribe long-term systemic antibiotics (tetra-cyclines or erythromycin). Apart from their action against bacteria, they have a special action on the cells in the lower layers of the skin to make them less likely to produce pustules. Minocycline is considered likely to be an effective treat-ment for moderate acne but more research is needed into acne treatments[18]. Dianette is a combined pill containing cyproterone acetate which reduces sebum production in the skin. It is also effective as a contraceptive. Dianette is only suitable for women because it works by lowering testosterone levels. The prescription must indicate the fact if Dianette is prescribed for contraception as well; otherwise the patient will have to pay a prescription charge.

Psoriasis

Psoriasis is a chronic skin condition with various types and degrees of severity. Arthritis is sometimes an associated condition. In the commonest plaque form, the disease is characterised by well-demarcated, scaly, dry, red patches. Topical treatments like coal tar and dithranol, although effective, can be messy, smelly and stain clothing. Calcipotriol is a non-staining ointment which may be more acceptable for treatment of plaque psoriasis. Emollients as bath additives and soap substitutes should be used every day to hydrate the skin.

Moderate sunlight may be beneficial, although sunburn can exacerbate the condition. Treatment with psoralens and ultraviolet light (PUVA) has been shown to be effective but can increase the risk of skin cancer. There may be periods of remission but the condition frequently flares up in response to stress or other trigger factors. Techniques for stress management may be helpful but have not been confirmed by enough research[19]. If steroid treatments are pre-scribed, their use should be monitored, because inappropriate long-term use can cause thinning of the skin. The finger-tip unit is a simple way of teaching patients how much cream or ointment to use to cover a given area[20].

Eczema

The terms eczema and dermatitis are essentially the same, and mean an inflammatory condition of the skin. The skin eruption may be red and weeping in acute eczema or thickened, dry and scaly in chronic stages. The rash usually causes severe itching and can be exacerbated by infection. There are several ways of classifying eczema:

- Allergic eczema is caused by sensitisation to an allergen such as nickel, lanolin, rubber or epoxy resins
- Irritant eczema occurs in response to substances like detergents, chemicals, or dusts (if eczema is related to the workplace the patient may need professional advice: information about occupational skin disease can be obtained from the Employment Medical Advisory Service[21])
- Atopic eczema usually starts in childhood and may accompany asthma and hay fever
- Seborrhoeic eczema – clearly defined red lesions with greasy scale, commonly occurs in the scalp, face and other parts of the skin with concentrations of sebaceous glands, and fungal infection is probably involved (HIV positive patients are particularly susceptible)
- Varicose eczema is secondary to venous insufficiency: can be exacerbated by allergic reactions to topical treatments
- Pompholyx eczema causes small vesicles on the palms and soles of the feet.

Treatment

Whatever the cause of eczema the treatments are often similar. In acute eczema povidone iodine or potassium permanganate soaks may be prescribed for their anti-infective effect and to dry weeping areas of skin. Systemic antibiotics will be required if the eczema is infected. Steroid creams will probably be needed to control the eczema, but should be avoided until any infection is treated because steroids can suppress the local immune response. Tar-based shampoo may be prescribed for treating seborrhoeic eczema by reducing sebum production, or antifungal preparations to treat fungal infections.

Long-term care requires diligent skin care and avoidance of exacerbating factors when possible. The evidence for many interventions is slim[22]. Evening primrose oil may have effective anti-inflammatory properties. Patients who choose to take Chinese herbal medicine should have regular liver function tests as they can be hepatotoxic.

The nurse can help to educate patients and others about the condition and provide support and practical advice on management. This will include:

- Hydration of the skin with emollient creams such as aqueous cream and emulsifying ointment, and unperfumed bath emollients (patients should be warned of the danger of slipping in a bath containing emollients, but bathing is a good way to hydrate the skin)
- Applying steroid creams correctly
- Avoiding soaps, perfumes and other irritants such as woollen clothing (cotton gloves can be worn inside rubber or plastic ones to protect the hands from contact)
- Providing information about the relevant support groups.

Cold sores (herpes simplex)

The common lesion caused by the herpes simplex virus is the unsightly cold sore. The virus is acquired, often as a child from the parent, and lives in the cells of the mucocutaneous junction of the lips. The virus proliferates when resistance is low, producing a tingling sensation followed by painful blisters. The blisters weep and crack and then form scabs which heal in about seven days. Once infected, recurrent attacks can occur in response to trigger factors like stress, sunlight, illness or pregnancy. The virus is contagious and can be spread to other people or to other parts of the body. Genital herpes, eye involvement and herpetic infection of eczema are some of the possible complications. Hence the need for education on ways of preventing spread of the virus by:

- Scrupulous hand hygiene
- Not kissing or engaging in oral sex when a cold sore is present
- Not sharing towels or utensils
- Not using saliva to moisten contact lenses.

Acyclovir cream, used early in the eruption, may help to minimise the effect. It needs to be applied every two hours, as soon as the tingling begins, to be of real benefit. Acyclovir cream can now be bought over the counter. Patients with genital herpes should usually be referred to the sexual health clinic for screening for other sexually transmitted diseases.

Boils and carbuncles

Infected hair follicles can develop into very painful swellings as a result of local inflammation and pus formation. Diabetes should always be ruled out because recurrent skin infections can be a presenting sign. Antibiotic treatment will be needed sometimes; but in many instances, after hot bathing, the lesion will discharge spontaneously, or be ready for incision. Carbuncles usually need incision, a light calcium alginate wick to encourage drainage, and dressings until healed.

Impetigo

Impetigo, a staphylococcal infection of the skin, can cause unsightly, weeping lesions, with a yellowish crust. The face is commonly affected. Muciprocin or fusidic acid ointment will usually clear the infection quickly, but strict personal hygiene (careful hand washing, and separate towels) is needed to prevent its being spread.

Fungal infections

Any part of the body may be affected by fungal infections, which can be treated with antifungal preparations. Babies can develop distressing fungal rashes in the napkin area. Scrupulous skincare is essential. Sometimes antifungal creams containing hydrocortisone are needed for a few days to treat the inflammation of the skin.

Athlete's foot (Tinea pedis)

Fungal infection readily occurs in the moist skin between the toes, causing itching, maceration and painful cracks. Left untreated, this can allow entry to other organisms, and result in severe infection of the legs and feet. Treatment with imidazole antifungal preparations (see *BNF*) is usually effective but ter-binafine (Lamisil) may be needed for intractable conditions and fungal nail infections. Recurrence is likely if patients do not follow these basic foot care measures:

- Wash the feet at least once a day and dry carefully between the toes (use antifungal treatment if athlete's foot is present)
- Wear clean socks or stockings every day
- Wear footwear which allows air to the feet
- Change footwear regularly
- See your doctor if the condition does not respond to treatment or the toenails become affected.

Warts

Warts are caused by different types of human papilloma virus. Warts on the hands and feet usually disappear spontaneously as the body develops immunity to the virus. Unfortunately this can take many months and patients with unsightly warts on the hands, or pressure symptoms from verrucae, are unlikely to want to wait. Plantar warts (verrucae) are very common in children but schools will sometimes try to exclude a child from swimming or games. Although unlikely to limit the spread, verruca socks can be worn to satisfy the school rules.

   If treatment is requested, topical preparations of salicylic acid can be recommended or prescribed. The manufacturer's instructions must be followed. The paint is applied daily, taking care to avoid the surrounding skin. A pumice stone or emery board must be used between applications to remove dead skin. Patients need to persevere with the treatment for up to six weeks. If there is no response minor surgery may be considered.

Genital warts

Genital warts are transmitted sexually (see Chapter 12, Sexual Health).

> ## Suggestions for reflection on practice
>
> Review your job description, professional education and experience.
>
> - Do you feel competent to deal with the medical conditions you encounter in your practice?
> - Do you have protocols to work to?
> - What further education/resources do you need?
> - How does your role as a nurse differ from that of a doctor or nurse practitioner in those instances?

Further reading

Greaves, B. (2000) Setting up nurse triage in practice. *Practice Nursing*, **11** (3), 20–2.

Johnson, G., Hill-Smith, I. & Ellis, C. (eds) (2000) *The Minor Illness Manual*, 2nd edition. Radcliffe, Oxon.

Royal College of Nursing (2000) *Nursing in NHS Walk-in Centres*. Royal College of Nursing, London.

References

1. Robinson, J. (2001) GPs' working patterns set for shake-up. *Pulse*, **61** (34), 1.
2. NHS (2001) *NHS walk-in centres. www.doh.gov.uk/nhswalincenres/info*
3. Parliament (1992) *The Medicinal Products: prescription by nurses etc. Act 1992*. HMSO, London.
4. Department of Health (Crown, J. Chair) (1999) *Review of Prescribing and Administration of Medicines final report*. HMSO, London
5. BNF (2001) Non-opioid analgesics, *British National Formulary*, **41**, 4.7.1.
6. Control of Substances Hazardous to Health regulations 1994 (COSHH).
7. British Society for Allergy and Clinical Immunology (2001) Rhinitis management guidelines. *Guidelines*, **14**, 323–8.
8. Bandolier (1995) *Antibiotics for Acute Otitis Media. www.jr2.ox.ac.uk/bandolier/band18/b16–3.html* (accessed 15/9/01).
9. McVerry, M. & Collin, J. (1999) Managing the child with gastroenteritis. *Nursing Standard*, **13** (37), 49–53.
10. Mead, M. (2000) Cystitis. *Practice Nurse*, **19**, 339–40.
11. Lavender, R. (2000) Cranberry juice: the facts. *Nursing Times Suppl. NTPlus*, **96** (40), 11–12.
12. Jepson, R. Mihaljevic, L. & Craig, J. (2001) Cranberries for treating urinary tract infections (Cochrane Review) *www.cochrane.org/cochrane/revabstr/ab001322* (accessed 9/9/01).
13. Kassianos, G. (2001) Varicella. In: *Immunisation Childhood and Travel Health*, 4th edn pp. 226–30.

14. British Infection Society (2001) Guidelines for the management of shingles. *Guidelines*, **14**, 191–2.

15. O'Morain, R. (13/7/2000) Measles epidemic with 1222 cases. *Irish Times*, front page.

16. NHS Centre for Reviews & Dissemination (1999) Treating head lice and scabies. *Effectiveness Matters*, 4, Issue 1.

17. Rolfe, G. (2001) Nurse-led skin clinics. *Practice Nurse*, **22** (4), 26–30.

18. Garner, S., Eady, A., Popescu, C., Newton, L. & Li Wan Po, A. (2001) *Minocycline for acne vulgaris: efficay and safety* (Cochrane Review) *www.cochrane.org/cochrane/revabstr/ ab002086* (accessed 9/9/01).

19. Naldi, L. (2000) Chronic plaque psoriasis. *Clinical Evidence*, **3**, 809–21. BMJ Publishing Group, London.

20. Long, C.C. & Finlay, A.Y. The finger-tip measure – a new practical measure. *Clinical and Experimental Dermatology*, **16**, 444–7.

21. Health and Safety Executive leaflet (2000) *The Employment Medical Advisory Service and You*. Health and Safety Executive, Sheffield.

Chapter 9
Health Promotion

Health promotion became a natural part of the practice nurse role when the GP Contract made general practice the focus for initiatives to promote healthy lifestyles and to prevent certain diseases. Various ways of reimbursing practices for health promotional activities were introduced and later dropped. Successive governments linked health promotion to targets outlined in their strategy documents. *The Health of the Nation* (1992) and *Saving Lives: Our Healthier Nation* (1998) were the English versions. Scotland, Wales and Northern Ireland produced similar strategies.

National Service Frameworks

Since 1999 a series of NSFs have been published. The first three cover mental health, coronary heart disease and older people; the NSF for diabetes is overdue. Every practice will have a copy of the NSFs and nurses are advised to familiarise themselves with them. It is envisaged that new ones will be published annually[1]. The NSF for coronary heart disease, published in March 2000, sets standards for the prevention and treatment of CHD and cardiac rehabilitation. The role within primary care of preventing CHD will be covered in this chapter but the reader should be aware of the wider medical and social issues.

Inequalities in health

It has long been recognised that poverty and lower social class have adverse effects on health. This was demonstrated by the Black report in 1980[2]. More recently the Acheson Report demonstrated that inequalities still exist[3]. Unskilled working men are three times more likely to die prematurely of CHD than men in professional or managerial occupations. Primary care organisations now produce health improvement programmes, which reflect the national and local priorities for improving health through collaboration between health and social care agencies and the public.

Cultural diversity

Britain is recognised as being multicultural. In terms of health promotion, this requires sensitivity to the needs of members of different cultural groups and an understanding of specific health needs. There may be a need for an interpreter, who is not a family member, or for literature in the appropriate language when English is not understood. Local health promotion or social service training departments usually provide sessions on cultural awareness to help nurses and doctors to examine their attitudes to members of other cultural groups and to develop strategies for meeting the needs of all their patients equitably.

Education for practice nurses

Practice nurses have accepted health promotion as a fundamental part of their work but they require a thorough understanding of the process and a good grounding in using models of health promotion in order to be truly effective. Training in negotiating behaviour change and motivational interviewing are recommended as a minimum for this role. Health promotion is also covered in depth on the community specialist (general practice nursing) degree courses. Good communication skills are a prerequisite for successful health promotion. Telling people what they ought to be doing is unlikely to succeed. Motivational interviewing is a way of helping people to recognise for themselves the need to change a risky behaviour and to decide on a suitable strategy for change.

Terminology

The term *health promotion* is used rather freely nowadays but its exact meaning warrants some reflection. *Health* is a complex issue; influenced as much by environmental, political, social and genetic factors as by personal behaviour or lifestyle. *Health promotion* is a broad term covering all those activities which contribute to the social, physical and mental well-being of individuals and societies. In general practice, it mainly involves preventive care and health education; although health workers may also campaign for action on the wider issues such as cigarette smoking shown on television or alcohol advertising at the cinema.

Prevention

Preventive care aims either to prevent ill health or to minimise its effect. Three types of prevention are recognised:

- *Primary Prevention* covers activities which aim to prevent disease from occurring, e.g. immunisation against infectious diseases, encouraging healthy eating and exercise.

- *Secondary Prevention* aims to detect problems before symptoms develop, in order to take early remedial action, e.g. child development checks, cervical and breast screening.

- *Tertiary Prevention* includes the management of existing disease or disability in order to minimise any complications and maximise the patient's quality of life, e.g. encouraging good glycaemic control in diabetes, controlling blood pressure to prevent heart failure or a stroke.

Screening entails looking for previously unrecognised disease in particular groups of people. Screening tests have to meet various criteria in order to be of value:

- The condition must be treatable
- It must develop slowly
- The test must be simple and reliable
- It must be cost-effective in terms of money and manpower[4].

No screening should be undertaken without informed consent. Patients could be subjected to unnecessary investigations and distress if screening tests produce false positive results. Conversely, false negative results may lead patients to ignore subsequent symptoms because of a false sense of security.

Health education

Health education seeks to provide learning opportunities about health, either by working with individuals or, generally, through the media or advertising. At the personal level, health education involves sharing knowledge about health, identifying any risks to health and helping people to develop the ability to make healthy choices.

Health promotion and the primary healthcare team

Nurses who undertake health promotion must have discussed the ethical implications and have a clear philosophy of health. Many health behaviours are highly complex, yet there is a danger of attributing blame to people whose actions are perceived as contributing to their own diseases. Health promotion activities should be evidence-based as far as possible by: seeking the existing evidence, collecting new evidence, questioning evidence and acting upon reliable evidence[5]. Doctors and nurses who 'practice what they preach' and act as role models for their patients may have greater credibility when offering advice to patients about healthy living.

Communication

Communication involves both the transmission and reception of information and ideas. Non-verbal communication relays messages, either consciously or unconsciously, through facial expression, gesture, general appearance and posture. All the senses pick up cues and confusion occurs when the non-verbal message conflicts with the spoken one.

A nurse should ensure that any information given is meaningful. Written material will be of little use if the patient is illiterate, cannot see well enough to read or does not understand the language in which it is written. Jargon can be a useful shorthand for those in the know but it is also a way of excluding out-siders. It follows that to use jargon to patients can exclude them as well. It is better to assume nothing and always check what the patient knows and has understood. Many of the techniques of counselling can be used in health promotion:

- *Suitable ambience*   A quiet, peaceful environment, free from telephone calls and visual distractions, will help concentration on the issues.

- *Asking open questions*   Closed questions such as, 'Do you drink any alcohol?' will elicit yes/no type answers. Open questions (often beginning with what, why, when, where or how) allow a subject to be explored, for example, 'How many days each week do you drink alcohol?' or 'What effect do you think this has on your health?'

- *Checking on understanding*   No matter how obvious the subject may seem to the nurse, it may be totally obscure to the patient; so it pays to take stock regularly. The nurse can ask the patient to recap in his/her own words what has been discussed. Alternatively, the nurse may paraphrase what the patient has said to make sure nothing has been misunderstood.

- *Active listening*   It requires a particular skill to be able to sit and give undi-vided attention to another person; to maintain a calm but attentive posture, to allow eye contact without staring, to give nods of encouragement when needed, but above all, to tolerate pauses without wanting to fill them.

Motivation

Knowledge about health risks alone will not cause people to alter their beha-viour. They must also feel motivated to change. This means that the rewards of change must outweigh the short-term benefits of the behaviour. Some patients are ambivalent; they want to change but are reluctant to give up the pleasures of their risky behaviour. *Motivational interviewing* is a technique developed by a psychologist to assist ambivalent people to decide to deal with addictive behaviour[6]. The key points involve:

- *Empathy*   Acceptance of the patient as a person. Trying to enter into the feelings of that person.

- *Developing discrepancy*   Helping the patient to decide to change and to pre-sent his/her own arguments for changing.

- *Avoiding confrontation*   Arguments are counterproductive.

- *Support for self-efficacy*   The patient is responsible for choosing and carrying out personal change.

Health promotion in general practice

Opportunistic health promotion can take place during any consultation or procedure; examples are given in other chapters. The remainder of this chapter deals with planned health promotion activities.

New patient health checks

The current GMS contract requires all new patients over five years of age to be offered a registration health check, to include measurement of height and weight, blood pressure and urinalysis for glucose and protein. Such interviews serve several purposes:

- Patients are welcomed to the surgery and given information about the services provided
- Essential points are ascertained about a patient's health before the NHS records are transferred (entries can be made to the appropriate disease registers)
- Doctors and nurses can gather details of a patient's social, medical and family history, identify potential health risks and offer appropriate help
- They attract an item of service fee.

Questionnaires can save some time but a face-to-face interview is also needed to clarify the information and to ensure that the patient consents to personal details being recorded. It is usual to record information on a computer, most of which have a selection of templates for health promotion. Sensitivity is required in interviewing, bearing in mind that the patient is in unfamiliar surroundings and may be feeling unwell. The questions need to be appropriate to the circumstances of individual patients. Close attention should be paid to the way questions are worded, as it would be very easy to give offence. There must be justifiable reasons for asking for information. Some of the information to be gathered is included under the following headings.

Social background

- *Title*   Ask how the patient would like to be addressed. (This can also elicit whether to address a woman as Mrs Miss or Ms; or if the patient has some other professional or honorary title.) Some patients deplore the modern trend towards addressing people by their first names.

- *Household* Ask if the patient has someone else at home. This might be a spouse or a partner, another relative or a lodger. It is wise to record the contact number and address of the person to be notified in an emergency, especially if the patient lives alone.

- *Carer* All new patients should be asked if they are caring for someone with a long-term physical or mental disability.

- *Children* The number and ages of any children may be relevant to the parent's health. A check can also be made on the immunisation status of children.

- *Employment* Check if there are any occupational hazards to consider. More ill-health and depression can occur in the unemployed[7]. If a woman has declared herself to be a housewife, it is insensitive to ask 'Do you work?' It is better to enquire about any work outside the home.

- *Smoking* Record if the patient has ever smoked. The quantity per day should be recorded in any smoking history and the year of stopping, if an ex-smoker.

- *Alcohol* If the patient is not teetotal ask how many units a day are consumed and how many days a week.

- *Exercise* Lack of exercise can be linked to many diseases. The frequency, duration and degree of any regular exercise undertaken should be recorded.

Past medical history

- *Illnesses* Any illnesses other than childhood infections should be noted.

- *Operations* List in chronological order.

- *Allergies* Some patients confuse allergies with side effects such as nausea, any true allergies must be documented prominently.

- *Immunisations* Patients who have not completed a full course against tetanus or polio can be offered immunisations; routine boosters are not required (see Chapter 10).

Current health

- *Current problems* Ask particularly about indigestion, pain, any abnormal bleeding or any problems with bladder or bowel function (consider the possibility of anaemia or thyroid dysfunction).

- *Medication* Ask what, if any, prescribed or OTC medicines are taken regularly.

Women

- *Obstetric history*   Ask about any pregnancies or miscarriages.

- *Periods*   Ask questions depending on the age of the patient – regularity of cycle, any problems, age at menopause, HRT.

- *Rubella status*   All women who could become pregnant should be immune to rubella and should be offered rubella antibody screening if appropriate.

- *Contraception*   Ask questions as appropriate. Check the method and need for further advice. If taking the pill, check for how many years. If they use an IUD or diaphragm, ask when it was last checked. If contraceptive injection, check when the next one is due. Ensure item of service claim is made.

- *Cervical smear*   If appropriate, record date and result of last smear, any history of abnormal smears/treatment. (Offer a smear appointment if it is due.)

- *Breasts*   Has the patient been taught breast awareness? Has she ever had mammography and if so, what was the result? (Offer advice or information if appropriate.)

- Use of HRT if post-menopausal.

Men

- *Testes*   Has the patient been taught about testicular self-examination? The incidence of testicular cancer in young men has been increasing and public awareness of the condition has been raised by high-profile campaigns in the media. TSE leaflets can be obtained from health promotion departments.

- *Prostate*   Ask about nocturia or any difficulty passing urine. Specific questions may detect problems which men attribute to ageing. Patients may wish to discuss testing for prostate cancer, which has been the focus of press attention recently. (See Chapter 14, Men's Health.)

Men can be diffident about expressing their feelings or concerns. They may be more willing to seek help when it is needed if a rapport is established during a new patient interview.

Family history

- *Parents and siblings*   Ask particularly about diabetes, CHD, hypertension, stroke, asthma, cancer, glaucoma, thyroid problems or tuberculosis: plus diagnosis and age at death (if no longer alive).

Tests

- *Height and weight*   Calculate the body mass index (weight in kilograms divided by the square of one's height in meters) from a BMI chart or computer programme. Check if the BMI is within the normal range (20–25 for men, 18.5–23.6 for women). Very muscular people may have a high BMI without having excess body fat.

- *Blood pressure*   Follow the practice protocol.

- *Urine (glucose)*   Screening for diabetes is a requirement of the GP contract but is not considered to be a reliable test for diabetes. A blood sugar test is needed if diabetes is suspected.

- *Urine (protein)*   Screen for renal disease or infection by testing for blood, nitrites and leucocytes or send an MSU if a urinary tract infection is suspected.

- *Peak expiratory flow rate*   Check this if there is a history of asthma.

Well-person checks

Patients may request a check-up at any time. Landmark birthdays, such as 40, 50 or 60 years, may trigger a sudden realisation of mortality. If a patient requests such a consultation, it is important to identify any particular health concerns and refer him/her to the doctor if necessary. Patients often have a vision of what a check-up should cover, which may be akin to the battery of tests and investigations undertaken by private health companies. Well-person health checks in general practice cover similar ground to that listed above (under new patient health checks). Although the emphasis may vary, depending on the age and sex of the patient. Lifestyle factors such as smoking, alcohol consumption, diet and exercise, together with blood pressure, BMI and family history, can be used to assess the risks for heart disease and to offer appropriate help. Various risk assessment tools are available, which can be used with caution in accordance with the practice protocol. One type can be found in the *British National Formulary*[8].

Assessment of older people

The GP contract requires all patients aged over 75 years to be offered an annual health check and home visit. Some practices still employ nurses to undertake this work, while others have found the results to be of limited value. The National Service Framework for Older People contains eight standards for ensuring that older people receive a consistently high level of service and are not denied access to healthcare because of age[9]. Systems are also required for ensuring that patients gain the maximum benefit from any medication and have their medication reviewed regularly. An over-75 health check can incorporate a medication review satisfactorily[10].

The NSF calls for the integration of assessment procedures for health and social care, which will entail cooperation between all the services involved and a rethinking of current assessment procedures. Practice nurses who undertake home visits must ensure that they have received appropriate education for the role. The extent of assessments would depend on local policies but the following points would usually be considered:

Social assessment

- *Housing* Check whether the patient lives in their own home, rented accommodation or sheltered housing.
  - Facilities (ask about toilet, bathing, cooking, heating)
  - Safety (ask about any loose rugs/floorboards, trailing flexes, unguarded fires)
  - Access (ask about stairs, lift, ground floor).

- *Carers* Check whether the patient lives alone, who is next of kin, level of support from family, friends, warden or social services, age of carers, or if the carers are on the register of carers. Do the carers need more support and is there evidence of tension in the household or of any abuse of the older person? (Elder abuse has been recognised as a serious problem in recent years[11].)

- *Finance* Is the patient able to keep the home warm, buy nutritious food, afford holidays or employ help if needed? Are all benefits being claimed, if entitled?

- *Lifestyle* Ask about smoking, alcohol consumption, nutrition, exercise, social contacts, clubs, hobbies.

Physical assessment

- *Ability to self-care* Ask how the patient manages cooking, bathing, shopping. Check the condition of their skin, hair and nails and ability to take any medication correctly.

- *Mobility* Ask about how they walk indoors and outdoors, and whether they manage stairs. Check which mobility aids they use and suitability of footwear.

- *Vision* Ask date of last eye check, and check use and condition of spectacles, and ability to read.

- *Hearing* Ask if they have any hearing impairment. If they use a hearing aid check their ability to use and maintain it.

- *Dentition* Ask about condition of teeth or dentures and whether they are able to visit a dentist if needed.

- *General health*   Ask about sleep, appetite, energy or any pain. Check for any signs of anaemia or thyroid dysfunction?

- *Continence*   Check whether there are any problems with bladder or bowel function and if continence aids/services are used or needed?

- *Tests*   Check blood pressure and urinalysis to detect hypertension, urinary tract infection or glycosuria.

- *Medication* (if taking any medicines)   Check whether the patient knows what they are for and when to take them. Ask if they were prescribed or OTC. Check they are still in date and whether any are duplicated with trade and generic names and if there is evidence of stockpiling.

Mental assessment

- *Level of consciousness*   Observe whether the patient is alert or drowsy and their ability to concentrate.

- *Mood*   Observe whether the patient appears normal, depressed, anxious or elated.

- *Thought and speech*   Note whether the patient's speech makes sense and any evidence of hallucinations or delusions.

- *Orientation and memory*   Check if the patient knows the date, where he/she lives, his/her age. Ask if the patient can remember what was said five minutes ago.

- *Behaviour*   Observe whether it appears appropriate to the circumstances.

A mental assessment can be more difficult than a physical assessment. Patients with early dementia can be very plausible and unless the nurse knows the family well, the problem may not always be apparent. A patient can give graphic details of his/her daily activities, which relate to years gone by and bear no relationship to the present situation.

Cautions   It would be wrong to assume that all older people are incapacitated in some way. As in every other generation, huge variations will be found. For every elderly, housebound person living in poverty, there will be another with a generous income, able to enjoy the freedom from work and family ties to travel and have fun.

Nurses should beware of promising help which cannot be delivered. False expectations can be aroused if situations are encountered for which there are few local services available. Loneliness and problems with bathing and foot-care are probably the most common problems but many social service and chiropody departments are overstretched. However, it would be pointless to carry out assessments of patients without acting upon any findings. Nurses must be aware of the procedure to follow if a problem comes to light. That will entail knowing:

- which health, voluntary or social services to contact
- when to refer to the GP or carry out further tests, e.g. blood sugar or thyroid function tests
- where to find information about private agencies or suppliers of equipment for patients who can afford them and wish to use them.

Dietary advice and monitoring

Dietitians are responsible for providing specialised dietary advice but practice nurses are usually expected to give guidance on healthy eating and to monitor patients on some diets. Collaboration allows the expertise of dietitians and nurses to be used effectively.

Healthy eating

Food is needed to provide the protein, vitamins and minerals required for healthy tissues and to supply the energy for daily activity and a normal body weight. Malabsorption, disease and anorexia can cause malnutrition but the majority of patients seeking advice are more likely to suffer from the effects of dietary excess. The incidence of obesity continues to rise despite the increased knowledge about its detrimental effects on health[12]. Most people would benefit from an increase in the consumption of complex carbohydrates and dietary fibre, and a reduction in fat, salt and sugar. Fruit and vegetables, pasta, rice and cereals should provide the greatest proportion of the diet with smaller quantities of protein and very little fat. The current thinking is that everyone should have at least five portions of fruit and vegetables a day[13].

Lipid-lowering diets

Patients are very aware of high cholesterol as a contributory factor for coronary artery disease. The *NSF for Coronary Heart Disease* expects 80–90% of people to be given a statin to lower their cholesterol level after a heart attack. Patients with an inherited hyperlipidaemia can also require treatment with lipid-lowering drugs.

The selection of asymptomatic patients for testing will depend on the practice policy, but talking to a patient who requests a cholesterol test will provide an opportunity for discussing other risk factors such as smoking, family history, raised BMI and lack of exercise. Help can be offered to consider appropriate lifestyle changes. Healthy eating and a control of dietary fat is beneficial for almost everyone. Less than 30% of the daily energy requirement should come from fat; of which not more that 10% should be saturated fat[14]. This will mean little to the average person, so it would be better to suggest reducing their total fat intake and replace animal fats such as full cream milk, butter and cheese with suitable low-fat alternatives by using low-fat spreads or those made with monounsaturated/polyunsaturated fats. Olive oil, sunflower oil, corn oil and low-fat oils and salad dressings could be discussed, with suggestions for cooking methods without the use of additional fat.

Patients may need to be reminded about hidden fats in cakes, biscuits and processed foods. The whole subject is a minefield and patients need to read food labels carefully if they are not to be misled by unrealistic claims on the packet. Pre-packed meals should not contain more than 5% fat, or more than 15 g fat per serving. Low-fat spreads and yoghourts vary considerably in their fat contents. Patients who do not need to lose weight will need to increase their intake of starchy food as they reduce their fats, in order to maintain their calorie intake. Patients should also be encouraged to use wholegrain products and increase their intake of oily fish, soluble fibre (oats and pulses), fruit and vegetables.

Weight loss

The cause of obesity is simple – more calories are consumed than the body uses for energy, so the excess is stored as fat. The complexity lies in the reasons for the mismatch. Very few people enjoy being overweight but strong psychological factors and ingrained behaviour affect their eating habits. There may even be genetic factors involved. Rapid weight loss can be followed by a rapid weight gain, as a result of metabolic changes. Therefore, the objective must be to help the patient to avoid drastic dieting and to substitute more suitable foods without creating an obsession with the next meal. The following steps can be helpful:

(1) *Obtain a full medical, social and family history*, to identify any factors which could affect the patient's weight.

(2) *Measure the current weight and height*, to calculate the body mass index and identify how much weight, if any, needs to be shed.

(3) *Assess the patient's motivation*, to find out if the patient wants to lose weight. Check if he/she perceives the increased risks of obesity to health (CHD, diabetes, osteoarthritis). Encourage the ambivalent patient to identify the personal benefits and positive reasons for change.

(4) *Identify the root cause of being overweight* instead of just dealing with the symptoms (i.e. by dieting).

(5) *Help the patient to set realistic goals*   Small steps, which can be reached in a reasonable time, will provide the encouragement to persevere. Success reinforces motivation.

(6) *Identify the patient's usual eating habits*   Ask the patient to keep an accurate food diary for at least a week. The diary should include the quantities as well as the types of food and drink and the circumstances when they were consumed. Alcohol consumption should also be recorded. Patients from other cultural backgrounds may eat foods with which the nurse is not familiar. The dietitian can be consulted about their nutritional values. Patients from developing countries may need to be persuaded to stick to their traditional foods and to avoid the high-fat hamburgers and foods full of salt or refined sugar so popular in western diets. However, some Asian patients may need to be persuaded to use cooking oil instead of ghee, which is mostly saturated fat, and to use less of it.

(7) *Negotiate changes to the diet*   Healthy eating will need to be lifelong. Drastic changes to eating habits will not be sustained if the patient does not like the substituted foods.

A nurse should be able to offer suggestions in accordance with the patient's income and religious beliefs. Sometimes compromises may be needed to help the patients to accept change. For example:

- *Milk*   If skimmed milk is unacceptable, try semi-skimmed. Skimmed milk can be used in some cooking, where it won't be tasted. If enough milk is not drunk each day low-fat yogurt will provide calcium and vitamins.

- *Salads*   Dieters who hate salads do not have to eat them. Alternatively, salad can be used in sandwiches, with hot food or after the main course, as they eat it in France. A teaspoonful of low-fat salad dressing can make all the difference to the taste of a salad.

- *Vegetables*   Several different vegetables, even if cooked in the same pot, will be more interesting than a plate loaded with one type. Jacket potatoes make a filling meal with cottage cheese, tuna, baked beans or yogurt with onions and herbs (instead of butter).

- *Fruit*   Tinned fruit in fruit juice can be found in most supermarkets. Dried fruits make a delicious snack. Fruits in season are cheaper than exotic imports, which carry high transport costs.

- *Meat*   It may be expensive but smaller quantities can be eaten. Lean meat, skinless chicken or low-fat sausages can be grilled, casseroled or baked, instead of fried. Poultry contains less fat but the skin must be removed before cooking.

- *Fibre*   If patients do not like wholemeal bread try high-fibre white bread as an alternative. A few chopped ready-to-eat dried apricots or raisins added to breakfast cereals will add sweetness and texture. If high fibre cereals are disliked, try mixing different cereals together to give variety and improve the taste.

(Any of the above examples could apply equally to patient who want to eat more healthily – even without losing weight.)

Once a patient has decided to lose weight the practice nurse can help by:

- *Monitoring progress* The rapid weight loss of the first weeks will slow down. Particular encouragement is needed when a plateau is reached. Increased physical activity can be advised and keeping a food diary can help to re-motivate the patient. New goals can be set as weight is lost. A good weight loss is 0.5–1 kg a week.

- *Dealing with lapses* Patients need to understand that relapses are a part of the cycle of change[15]. If the patient wishes to lose weight then he/she can begin again by planning how to deal with difficult situations and instead of feeling like a failure, have a positive attitude to change.

- *Encouraging maintenance of the target weight* Once the patient has reached the final goal, adjustments to the diet will need to be made to stay at the target weight. Euphoria at having achieved the goal can lead the patient to resume the old habits of eating. Throughout the period of weight loss, the benefits of permanent change must be stressed. Binge eating at this important stage of the process could be disastrous.

Discussions about diet should be accompanied by recommendations for appropriate exercise and sensible drinking.

Exercise

It is now possible in some areas to prescribe exercise in a similar way to pre-scribing drugs, and arrangements have been made with local leisure centres for patients to take part in structured exercise. Even more innovative schemes have been reported, such as the *green gym* which links exercise to conservation work[16]. Physical activity has many benefits for health; not least in the pre-vention of coronary heart disease and diabetes. The level of activity must be appropriate for each individual patient. Advice booklets can be obtained from the health promotion department. Patients who are very obese or have a history of hypertension or heart disease may require specific advice from a physio-therapist.

Sensible drinking

Alcohol consumption is an important part of any health assessment. People of all ages have ready access to drink and millions of workdays are lost each year through drink-related absenteeism. Measurements in units of alcohol make assessment easier, providing that patients understand what constitutes a unit and give an accurate report of their consumption. One unit, equivalent to 8 g of pure alcohol, is found in:

- 1/2 pint of ordinary strength beer
- 1 single pub measure of spirits
- 1 small glass of wine.

Therefore, a patient who drinks an aperitif each evening and half a bottle of wine with dinner is likely to be drinking 5–6 units daily. Sensible drinking is considered to be below 28 units a week for men and 21 units for women spread evenly over the week[17]. Patients should be made aware that drinking all recommended units at a weekend can be more harmful than drinking regular daily amounts. They also need to know that drinking more than the recommended amount can have adverse effects on health, particularly the liver. Alcohol in pregnancy or while breastfeeding can be damaging to the fetus/baby. So women must be advised not to have more than a very occasional drink in those circumstances.

Patients who answer 'yes' to two or more questions in the CAGE questionnaire are more likely to be dependent on alcohol:

(1) Have you ever felt you should **C**ut down on your drinking?
(2) Have people **A**nnoyed you by criticising your drinking?
(3) Have you ever felt bad or **G**uilty about your drinking?
(4) Have you ever had a drink in the morning to steady your nerves or get rid of a hangover (**E**ye-opener)?

The use of this or other short questionnaires, together with full blood count and liver function tests, will detect a high percentage of people with a serious alcohol problem[18].

Patients with alcohol dependence, who are willing to be helped, may require medical supervision or a support service such as Alcoholics Anonymous. Practice nurses can help patients who want to drink less to agree on a sensible limit and devise strategies for sticking to it. However, this is dependent on the nurses themselves having the necessary knowledge and there is some evidence that some nurses and doctors need more education about the subject[19].

A drink diary can help the patient to stay within the target limit and to recognise the times and situations when the pressure to drink is greatest. Ways of cutting down which may be adopted include:

- Keep busy to avoid thinking about drink
- Postpone the first drink until as late as possible in the day
- Drink halves instead of pints
- Try low alcohol drinks instead
- Dilute spirits with mixers
- Take small sips and make a drink last
- Don't get involved in buying rounds – it can involve trying to keep pace with other drinkers

- Use a measure at home to make sure a drink is only a single, then put the bottle out of sight.

The relationship between drinking and social activities can vary. The importance of not drinking and driving can make the refusal of alcohol more socially acceptable, but in other circumstances peer pressure can be very strong. Sadly, a lot of alcohol advertisements seem to be aimed at young people. The money spent persuading them to drink far outweighs the resources available for health education, despite some very good initiatives by schools and school nurses.

Smoking cessation

There is an increasing public awareness of the health risks from smoking and pressure on smokers to quit. Health workers are required to identify the patients who smoke, explain the dangers to health and to provide access to services to help them stop smoking[20]. Nicotine replacement products or the drug buproprion can be prescribed, when appropriate, together with quit-smoking counselling to help patients to overcome the addiction to nicotine. Some practice nurses have undergone the training needed for the role of smoking cessation counsellor. This work is also being taken on by pharmacists in some areas. Practice nurses should be aware of local arrangements and the support services for people who want to stop smoking. If a patient is ambivalent about quitting, the health professional has a duty to ensure that he/she has the facts about smoking and knows that help is available whenever the time is right to stop. No one can force a patient to quit; it must be a personal decision.

The dangers of smoking to health

These include:

- Heart disease and hypertension
- Peripheral vascular disease
- Chronic obstructive pulmonary disease
- Cancer of the lung, throat, mouth, tongue
- Cancer of the stomach, pancreas, cervix
- Pregnant women are more likely to have smaller, unhealthy babies
- Children who live in an environment where people smoke are more likely to have respiratory problems.

Patients will sometimes have symptoms of these conditions before they will accept help. They must be assured that it is never too late to give up smoking and that it can be a very important way of improving health. It is important to understand the social and psychological pressures which lead people to take up smoking and to avoid being judgemental. Parents need to be aware that children learn by example and are statistically more likely to start smoking if they come from a home where people smoke. Particular emphasis is being placed on helping pregnant mothers to quit smoking.

Helping patients quit smoking

A carbon monoxide monitor and/or a spirometer can be useful tools for convincing patients of the effects of smoking. A patient who wants to quit can be helped to devise a plan:

(1)   Work out all the reasons for stopping
(2)   Decide a date to stop, avoiding a day likely to be stressful
(3)   Tell people in close contact of the decision and try to persuade someone else to quit at the same time – for mutual support
(4)   Decide how to change the routine to avoid the usual triggers for smoking
(5)   Have nicotine replacement products ready, if needed, and contact details of support person or organisation
(6)   The evening before the quit day smoke the last cigarette and then throw away any remaining cigarettes.

Hints for the new non-smoker

- Avoid temptation – put ashtrays, matches and lighter out of sight
- Keep away from smokers (if possible)
- Change habits – avoid breaks when a cigarette is usually smoked
- Keep busy
- Put aside the money saved each day, for a reward for perseverance later on
- Keep a supply of chewing gum, apple or carrot to nibble if necessary
- Take more exercise to avoid gaining weight.

Suggestions for reflection on practice

- Consider your role in health promotion.
- How do you measure success?
- Could anything be done differently?

Further reading

Department of Health (2000) *No Secrets: Guidance on developing and implementing multi-agency policies and procedures to protect vulnerable adults from abuse.* Department of Health, London.

NHS Centre for Reviews and Dissemination (1998) Smoking cessation: what the health service can do. *Effectiveness Matters*, **3**, 1.

Perkins, E. Simnett, I. & Wright, L. (1999) *Evidence-Based Health Promotion*. Wiley, Chichester.

References

1. Department of Health. National Service Frameworks. *www.doh.gov.uk/nsf/about*
2. Townsend, P., Davidson, N. & Whitehead, M. (1988) *Inequalities in Health: The Black Report and The Health Divide*. Penguin Books, Harmondsworth.
3. Acheson, D. (1998) *Independent Enquiry into Inequalities in Health Report*. HMSO, London.
4. Larson, E. (1986) Evaluating the validity of screening tests. *Nursing Research*, **35** (3), 186–8.
5. Perkins, E.R., Simmett, I. & Wright, L. (1999) Creative tensions in evidence-based practice. In: *Evidence-Based Health Promotion*. Wiley, Chichester.
6. Miller, W. & Rollnick, S. (eds) (1991) *Motivational Interviewing: preparing people to change addictive behaviour*. Guildford Press, London.
7. Shortt, S. (1996) Is unemployment pathogenic? A review of current concepts with lessons for policy planners. *International Journal of Health Services*, **26** (3), 569–89.
8. Joint British Societies Coronary Risk Prediction Chart (2001) In: *British National Formulary*, 41, British Medical Association and Royal Pharmaceutical Society, London.
9. Department of Health (2001) *National Service Framework for Older People*. HMSO, London.
10. Lowe, C., Raynor, D., Teale, C. & Lubgan, C. (2000) Can practice nurses identify medication problems using the over-75 health check? *Journal of Clinical Nursing*, **50**, 172–5.
11. Hoban, S. & Kearney, K. (2000) Elder abuse and neglect. It takes many forms – if you're not looking for it you may miss it. *American Journal of Nursing*, **100** (11), 49–50.
12. Department of Health (1998) *Health Survey for England*. HMSO, London.
13. Health Education Authority (1994) *The Balance of Good Health Plate*. Health Education Authority, London.
14. Department of Health (1991) *The Health of the Nation*. HMSO, London.
15. Prochaska, J. & Di Clemente, C. (1989) Transtheoretical therapy: toward a more interpretative model of change. *Psychotherapy: Theory, Research and Practice*, **20**, 161–73.
16. Reynolds, V. (2000) What happened down at the green gym. *Practice Nurse*, **20** (9), 520–23.
17. Department of Health (1995) *Sensible Drinking. The report of an inter-departmental working group*. HMSO, London.
18. Aertgeerts, F., Buntinx, F., Ansoms, S. & Fevery, J. (2001) Screening properties of questionnaires and laboratory tests for the detection of alcohol abuse or dependence in a general practice setting. *British Journal of General Practice*, **51**, 206–17.
19. Webster-Harrison, P., Barton, A., Barton, S. & Anderson, S. (2001) General practitioners' and practice nurses' knowledge of how much people should and do drink. *British Journal of General Practice*, **51**, 218–20.
20. Parliament (1998) *Smoking Kills: a White Paper on Tobacco*. HMSO, London.

Useful address and web site

Health Promotion England
50 Eastbourne Terrace, London W2 3QR
Telephone: 020 7725 2880 Fax 020 7725 2881
Web site *www.hpe.org.uk*

Chapter 10
Child Health, Childhood and Adult Immunisation

Written by Veronique Gibbons
Immunisation Advice Nurse, PHLS

Child health surveillance

The GP Contract (1990) allows remuneration to GP for child health surveillance of the under-fives, and target payments for childhood immunisations. Prior to this, these services were commonly thought to be the work of health visitors[1]. In this context *surveillance* refers to normal growth and development. The purpose of such checks is to detect any problems early, so remedial action can be taken as soon as possible.

The family has input from many members of the primary health care team in the first months. The GP or midwife will perform the neonatal examination. The health visitor will establish contact with the family and assess the family's probable health needs. The 6–8 week check, performed by the GP, is to detect those disorders that do not always manifest at birth, for example, some types of congenital heart disease. If performed at two months of age, this examination coincides with a child's first primary immunisation course. The eight-month check is an ideal time for the distraction test and at 21 months, children with severe developmental or growth problems can be detected. Some areas vary in the ages at which these tests are performed and all checks are listed in the personal child health record (PCHR).

Child health surveillance has many aims but few of these services are evaluated. With clinical governance, a service based on teamwork, leadership, audit, patient involvement, evidence-based clinical methods, sharing and examining of both good practice and learning from mistakes can help develop a quality service[2].

Note Parents who see the word surveillance in records or on the computer screen, can be shocked if they think it means their child is on the at-risk register. A practice nurse may be asked for information, so it can help to be familiar with the specific practice arrangements and to have observed developmental checks being carried out.

At birth

Screening of the newborn is important, as most major abnormalities, syndromes, conditions etc. that can affect children are identified at this time. One examination in the first 36 hours is sufficient and is usually performed by a paediatrician prior to discharge from hospital[3]. A brief history of the health of the parents, of this pregnancy, of previous pregnancies and of brothers and sisters is taken. Any antenatal problems are identified. Any history of congenital heart disease, dislocation of the hips and hearing loss should be talked about, as parents may have anxieties about these.

Every baby has a full medical examination in the neonatal period. While the baby is asleep, posture, colour and respiratory rate can be observed. Listening to the heart for murmurs while the baby is asleep or quiet is easier than when it has just been woken. The head circumference is measured, while also observing the fontanelles and the face. The eyes are checked for conjunctivitis or cataracts and the pupils are examined. The nose is also examined, in particular to ensure that the nares are patent (choanal atresia causes respiratory distress – the skin looks pink when resting but blue when crying or feeding). The mouth is checked by palpating and visualising the palate to exclude clefts, as well as assessing the neck for lumps and the nipples for mastitis (as a result of maternal hormones).

The abdomen is palpated, including checks for hernias and whether meconium was passed in the first 24 hours. Limbs are assessed for symmetry and the hips for signs of congenital dislocation. Head circumference, weight and length may be recorded in the PCHR. A heel-prick blood test is performed by the midwife to check for congenital hypothyroidism and phenylketonuria; both of which can cause learning disabilities if not detected.

At ten to twenty-one days

A health visitor assessment is done but a physical examination is not required if the child has had a neonatal examination. If no neonatal examination has been performed, the child must be examined by their GP. During this examination head circumference is taken (often more accurate than the measurement at birth), eyes, mouth, umbilicus, testes in boys, muscle tone, skin, colour, heart murmur, hearing and vision are assessed. Oral vitamin K may have been given at birth instead of IM and the health visitor will need to remind the mother to give two further doses, at one week and four weeks if the child is mainly breastfed. No further doses are required if the child is mainly formula fed. This is also an opportune time to assess how the mother is coping, assessing for maternal depression and neglect or abuse. No opportunity should be missed for health promotion such as information about Sudden Infant Death Syndrome, passive smoking, feeding, immunisation, and safety (at home and in cars).

At six to eight weeks

The GP reviews the pregnancy and family history and discusses any concerns with the parents. A full physical examination, including hips and testes, is carried out and the baby's motor development is tested. Late detection of undescended testes is a problem and surgical correction before the age of 18 months is desirable because of the better chance of fertility. The weight, length and head circumference are measured and the hearing and vision assessed. Normally children show a startle response to a sudden noise and can follow a moving object with the eyes, to 90° on the horizontal. The practice will have its own arrangements for sharing developmental monitoring between the GP and the health visitor. There may be local variations in the timing of checks and in the professionals who actually perform them.

At eight months

Any parental concerns, especially about vision and hearing are discussed and the motor development is assessed. At this age, a child will enjoy peek-a-boo games. A distraction hearing test is performed, and the eyes are observed for squint or other possible problems with vision. Health promotion focuses around accident prevention, nutrition, dental care, safety in cars, passive smoking, developmental needs, sunburn and iron deficiency, if necessary.

At eighteen months to two years

The development of language and walking are assessed. A referral is needed for specialised testing at any age if there are any doubts about a child's vision, hearing or attainment of milestones in development. Health promotion focuses on developmental needs, language and play. At this age the child would benefit from mixing with other children. Discussion is usual about toilet training and their first dental appointment.

The Checklist for Autism in Toddlers (CHAT) has been successfully used to detect autism in a large community study of 16 000 children at 18-months-old[4]. CHAT consists of a questionnaire for the parent and a series of related and confirmatory observations for the health visitor. Children with autism may show abnormalities of both functional play, which is using objects as they are intended to be used, and sensorimotor play, which is banging them. Autism is difficult to differentiate from severe learning difficulty in children.

At three and a half years

Any parental concerns are discussed and a physical examination carried out as necessary. The height and weight are recorded. Tests are performed of language, gross motor and fine motor development, vision and hearing. The tests are incorporated in activities, which are presented as games to the child.

Assessments by the doctor or health visitor are made at other ages as well. All the staff should be alert to anything that seems amiss whenever a child is seen in the surgery. A practice nurse might be as concerned about a child who seems unduly passive during a treatment, as about one that wreaks absolute havoc in the treatment room. Teachers and school nurses may report any developmental problems once a child is at school.

Inherited conditions

A child who may have inherited a condition such a sickle cell disease, thalassaemia, or cystic fibrosis may be referred for testing, so that early prophylactic measures can be taken. The rapid growth in the technology has made genetic screening possible and the development of gene therapy provides hope for the future.

A practice nurse's main involvement in child health clinics may consist of giving the immunisations but parents will often ask for advice or information about other issues. Opportunities for health promotion should not be overlooked.

Safety

All adults have a duty to try and prevent accidents and injury to children. *Saving Lives: Our Healthier Nation* has a target for reducing the death rate by a fifth and serious injury caused by accidents by at least a tenth by the year 2010. Advice can be provided on:

- The safe storage of medicines and chemicals in the home and the use of childproof bottle tops and cupboard-closing devices
- Potential hazards such as stairs, furniture, windows, balconies, cookers, fires, electricity; and how to make them safer
- Potentially dangerous toys and games
- The risk to health from lack of exercise
- Road safety, safety seats in cars, and protection for cyclists
- How to avoid personal danger, or get help if abused.

The prevention of coronary heart disease and lifestyle-related illness needs to begin early. Children and adolescents are particularly susceptible to pressure from their peers to experiment with smoking, alcohol, drugs or solvents. A practice nurse can sometimes initiate discussions on these health issues, and be a source of information about the help and services available for worried parents and young people. Joint initiatives with school nurses and health visitors can help to ensure that a consistent message is being put across and nurses can also act as a pressure group. If hundreds of nurses telephone the television company to complain every time an actor lights a cigarette in a play on TV, it might be more effective in the long run than exhorting young people not to smoke.

Developing sexuality is another major concern for teenagers. Nurses with the appropriate training have an important role in promoting sexual health. The guarantee of confidentiality might encourage more teenagers to seek advice on sexual behaviour and contraception, although many of them are reluctant to visit the surgery, fearing that their parents will be informed. In some areas, community nurses are successfully running services in youth clubs and less formal settings[5].

Child abuse

A practice nurse could be the first person to whom a parent discloses information regarding the exposure of themselves or their children to physical or mental abuse. The parent may be scared and not wish to report such incidents. At this point it is important that the practice nurse is aware of local child protection policy. Every district has a formal child protection policy and staff in general practice must be aware of the procedure to follow. Most primary care trusts/community trusts hold regular training on child protection, which practice nurses should attend. By knowingly keeping a child in a risk situation there may be neglect in the nurse's duty of care, relating to the Children Act (1989). Not sharing concerns may amount to collusion. This is an extremely sensitive area in which one must act quickly.

The practice nurse could be the first to suspect physical or mental abuse to a child. Any abnormal or frequent injuries; particularly those with special significance, such as small circular burns (cigarettes), bruises suggestive of fingertip grasps on the upper arms, or from blows to the ears and lips. The relationship between the child and parent should also be noted. The rise in cases of recognised and reported child sexual abuse has highlighted an area in which doctors and nurses have to be particularly vigilant. Any suggestion of sexual abuse, from physical findings, verbal comments or behaviour, must be taken seriously. It is important to deal with these matters confidentially and sensitively. Producing definite evidence is often extremely difficult.

Because of the close relationship with the patients, a practice nurse will be familiar with the background and problems of many local families and be aware of those at risk from factors such as poverty, stress or alcoholism. It should be borne in mind that the incidence of abuse covers all social classes and income groups not just the socially deprived.

The Children Act (1989)

The Children Act gathered all the existing legislation relating to children into a new unified law. Many aspects of the Children Act concern child protection.

The child's welfare should be the paramount consideration at all times. This overrides the concern for the welfare of adults or carers, or concern about the future of the professional relationship. Health professionals have specific duties laid out in *Working Together*[6], and local procedures. Social services have a duty to investigate all children in their area, where there is a suspicion that a child is suffering or likely to suffer significant harm. Once a problem is identified and the decision to refer is taken, confidentiality has to be breached, as this will be in the child's best interest, regardless of the parent's disagreement.

Practice nurses should be aware that any child regardless of age, considered mature enough to understand all the issues, might give or withhold his/her own consent for treatment. The Department of Health has recently published guidelines relating to consent for children and young people[7].

Childhood and adult immunisation

Organisation

The GP Contract identified targets for childhood immunisations. The GP will be eligible for a full target payment if, on the first day of a quarter the number of courses completed in each of the groups of immunisations of all the children aged two on the partnership list on that day amounts, on average, to 90% of the number of courses needed to achieve full immunisation. Likewise they will receive a lower level of payment if the average of courses completed amounts to 70% of the number needed for full immunisation. For the purpose of target payments, immunisations fall into four groups (children aged two):

- Group 1 diphtheria/tetanus/poliomyelitis – 3 doses
- Group 2 pertussis – 3 doses
- Group 3 measles/mumps/rubella – 1 dose
- Group 4 Haemophilus influenza type B – 3 doses or a single dose after the age of 13 months.

Targets were introduced to improve immunisation uptake and therefore, reduce the spread of childhood communicable diseases. In order to do this, a monetary incentive was offered to GPs. The achievement of immunisation targets involves all the practice team and the calculation of targets takes into account immunisations carried out by others, including health authority clinics. Alongside this is the collection of information relating to the percentage of children in an area who have received vaccinations. Immunisation statistics, known as Coverage of Vaccinations Evaluated Rapidly (COVER), identify pockets of susceptibility within a community and focus on services within these areas. This also enables epidemiologists to analyse whether potential outbreaks may occur as a result of a drop in coverage.

Medico-legal aspects of immunisation

Any nurse undertaking immunisation needs to be familiar with the Green Book – *Immunisation against Infectious Disease*[8]. This valuable publication was due to be updated in 2002 by the Department of Health and the Public Health Laboratory Service. One copy is distributed to GP surgeries, but this may change with the updated version, which may be available electronically. It specifies the conditions under which nurses are covered to give immunisations. Each area will have local guidelines and for nurses, patient group directions (PGDs) will enable specified nurses the right to administer prescription only medications without an individual prescription from a doctor[9]. Most commonly PGDs will cover vaccinations in the national immunisation programme and for foreign travel. An extension to this may include medications for chronic diseases, such as asthma. The law restricts the use of PGDs to the NHS or organisations providing care for NHS patients as part of a contract with the NHS. Nurses using PGDs in non-NHS settings should seek guidance from their professional organisation or insurer.

Criteria for nurses

Nurses must fulfil three criteria:

- To be willing to be professionally accountable
- To have received specific training and be competent in all aspects of immunisation, including contraindications to specific vaccines
- To have had adequate training in dealing with anaphylaxis.

Consent

Consent can be written, oral or non-verbal. A signature on a consent form does not itself prove the consent is valid. If a nanny or anyone other than the parent or legal guardian brings a child for immunisation the nurse must ensure that their consent has been obtained. Local trusts should have a policy on when a nurse needs to obtain written consent. Consent must be given voluntarily, not under any form of duress or undue influence from health professionals, family or friends. Children under the age of 16, who are considered to be competent under the Gillick ruling, may give their own consent to immunisation[10].

Injection sites

The PGD should specify the preferred sites for immunisation, in conjunction with the manufacturer's instructions for specific vaccines. The Green Book takes into account recommendations that reflect present national immunisation policy. With the exception of BCG, oral typhoid and oral polio vaccines, all vaccines should be given intramuscularly or by deep subcutaneous injection.

Considerations should be given to the correct method of administration in people with coagulopathies.

In general, infants under one year of age should receive all vaccines in the antero-lateral aspect of the thigh; over the age of one, in the antero-lateral aspect of the thigh or deltoid; and for older children and adults, the deltoid is recommended. The buttock is not used because of the risk of sciatic nerve damage and it has been shown to reduce the efficacy of some vaccines, e.g. hepatitis B[11].

Emergency situations

Anaphylaxis is a rare occurrence, but it should always be anticipated. Adrenaline and basic resuscitation equipment must be available. The decision on whether to give immunisations without a doctor being on the premises will depend on the practice policy, plus the individual nurse's experience and willingness to accept the responsibility. Given the potential for tragedy, caution seems sensible. A plan of action for emergencies is essential, whether giving immunisations in the surgery or in patients' homes. The guidelines for the administration of adrenaline (epinephrine) changed in March 2001 to reflect its use in the community and the use of adrenaline pens. Practice nurses need to keep up to date with new guidelines while ensuring their skills are updated regularly (see Chapter 7 under anaphylaxis).

Childhood immunisation schedule

The primary course of immunisation is given at two, three and four months of age. This consists of:

- Combined diphtheria, tetanus, and pertussis vaccine (DTP) and *Haemophilus influenzae* type B vaccine (Hib)
- Meningitis C vaccine (MenC)
- Oral polio vaccine (OPV).

Inactivated polio vaccine may be given if live virus vaccine (OPV) is contraindicated. Fewer reactions have been noted in children who have had acellular pertussis vaccine when they have previously had a reaction from whole-cell pertussis vaccine. However, the acellular vaccines currently available may not provide the same degree of protection against pertussis as the whole-cell vaccine[12]. Pertussis vaccine may be contraindicated for some children who have ongoing neurological involvement; diphtheria/tetanus vaccine (DT) should be given in its place. These children will be susceptible to pertussis infection but as they get older their risk from the effects of pertussis is reduced. It is worth noting, however, that they will be able to pass on the virus to other susceptible individuals and this is just one of the reasons that herd immunity is so important. This is a level at which communicable diseases cannot be transmitted due to a high level of immunity in the environment.

Later courses of immunisation consist of:

- At 12–18 months mumps, measles and rubella vaccine (MMR) is due
- At 3.5–5 years pre-school reinforcing dose of diphtheria and tetanus and acellular pertussis (DTaP), oral polio (OPV) and a further MMR are given to children. Three years should elapse between the third DTP and the pre-school booster but a second dose of MMR can be given three months after the first. Meningitis C vaccine should be given if missed out previously. Hib is not given after the age of four unless there are other indications such as asplenia or haemaglobinopathies.

Acellular pertussis with diphtheria and tetanus (DTaP) became the vaccine for use in pre-school boosters from November 2001; replacing the DT vaccines used previously. The reason for the change is to protect infants, who are too young to be fully protected, from catching pertussis transmitted by older siblings, as well as to protect older children from the disease[13].

Efficient organisation is needed, whether the call/recall system for immunisation is centrally administered or one devised by the individual practice. Birthday cards at strategic dates can provide friendly reminders:

- One year for MMR
- Four years for pre-school boosters
- Fifteen years for tetanus/low dose diphtheria and polio boosters. (MMR should also be considered for those adolescents who did not have an MMR and were given one dose of measles/rubella (MR) during the November 1994 catch up campaign, thus missing out on mumps immunity. As is now evident with recent mumps outbreaks amongst teenagers, the incidence has moved to an age group who are still susceptible.)

Opportunistic immunisation can be aided by flagging the records of patients. Flexible timing of appointments can help, but home visiting may sometimes be necessary; immunisation at home may be undertaken by the health visitor.

Contraindications to immunisation

Many conditions previously thought to contraindicate immunisation, such as asthma, no longer apply. Immunisation should be postponed if the patient has any acute febrile illness. A severe local or general reaction to a previous dose would be a definite contraindication to further administration of the same vaccine, until further advice is sought. Such reactions need to be differentiated from the milder reactions that can often be expected to occur. No child should be denied the protection of immunisation without very good cause.

Live virus vaccines are generally contraindicated for:

- Immunocompromised patients such as those receiving high-dose steroids and patients with malignant conditions or other diseases affecting their immune systems, such as HIV
- Pregnant women
- Patients who have received another live vaccine within the past three weeks, unless given simultaneously.

The details about specific immunisations and their contraindications are not repeated here, because the Green Book provides such comprehensive information. The nurse must be sure that there are no contraindications to a specific vaccine being given. A medical opinion should be requested when necessary.

Information for parents

Written information is useful to reinforce verbal advice about possible reactions and how to deal with them. Infant paracetamol is usually recommended for fever or prolonged crying and this is given at a dose of 10–15 mg/kg body weight (maximum of 60 mg). The dose varies between products. (See British National Formulary.) The paracetamol products are licensed for treating infants under three months of age for post-immunisation fever. Parents should know how to get medical help if worried and be asked to report any severe reactions. DPT vaccine can cause a harmless lump, about the size of a small pea, under the skin. This is usually due to the vaccine being given too shallowly, although research suggests that the use of a longer needle reduces the incidence of adverse reactions[14]. Any reaction from MMR usually follows the incubation time of the actual diseases. Thus mild symptoms of measles may occur from 7–12 days, possibly with fever and a rash. Mumps takes slightly longer (14–21 days). There may be slight fever and parotid swelling. These reactions are non-infectious, so the children do not need to be isolated.

Other immunisations

Tuberculosis

Bacillus Calmette-Guérin vaccine (BCG) is a live, attenuated, freeze-dried vaccine not usually given in general practice. In high-risk areas infants may be immunised at birth; otherwise children aged 10–13 receive BCG through the school health service. Parents planning long-term travel to countries with a high incidence of tuberculosis should be advised to consider BCG immunisation for their children. Usually a referral from the GP to the local chest clinic will be sought. Special training is required to administer BCG vaccines and skin tests. Poor technique can result in unsightly scars.

Special risks

Occasionally immunisation may be needed to protect children at particular risk from contact with hepatitis B, or from influenza or pneumococcal infections which could complicate other medical conditions (see the Green Book). Since April 2000, women have been screened for hepatitis B status antenatally to reduce the high rate of chronic carrier state from natural passive transmission which is 70–90% in babies under the age of one year. Infants born to hepatitis B positive mothers begin immunisation as soon as possible after birth.

Adult immunisation

The immunisation of adults may be performed for the following reasons:

- Missed or incomplete childhood immunisations (vaccines may not have been available then)
- Special risk of exposure through injury, occupation, health status, or lifestyle
- Reinforcing doses are required to maintain immunity.

Tetanus immunisation

Routine immunisation against tetanus was introduced in 1961, although it was given to people in the armed forces before then. Therefore, patients born before that date, who did not serve in the armed forces, may never have been immunised. They require a primary course of adsorbed tetanus vaccine, three doses of 0.5 ml by intramuscular (IM) or deep subcutaneous (SC) injection at monthly intervals, a booster five years later and a further reinforcing dose ten years afterwards. Any unfinished course may be completed at any time without restarting a new course. Once an individual has received five tetanus injections, boosters are only recommended if a tetanus-prone wound is sustained or if travelling to a country where hygienic immunisation practices may not be guaranteed. Unnecessary booster doses can result in severe local reactions.

Poliomyelitis immunisation

Patients born before 1958 may not have been immunised against polio. Any unimmunised adult should be offered the vaccine. Unless contraindicated, three doses of oral polio vaccine should be given at monthly intervals. Inactivated vaccine may be used if live virus is contraindicated. Reinforcing doses are not required, unless at special risk from foreign travel or occupational exposure.

Poliovirus can be excreted in the faeces for about six weeks after immunisation. Parents who were not fully immunised should be offered polio vaccine at the same time as their babies, and be warned about careful hand washing after nappy changing. This is different from previous advice of routinely giving parents OPV regardless of immunisation status when presenting with an infant for immunisation. Human normal immunoglobulin is used when OPV is inadvertently given which puts a patient or a contact at risk of contracting polio, e.g. immunocompromised. This can be obtained from the Public Health Laboratory Service.

Rubella immunisation

It is hoped that the immunisation of all children with MMR will eventually remove the main pool of rubella infection. All women of childbearing age should be screened for rubella antibodies and immunised if necessary. A single dose of rubella vaccine 0.5 ml by SC or IM injection is required. The date of the LMP should be ascertained because rubella immunisation should not be given if pregnancy is a possibility. Women should also be advised not to become pregnant for at least one month after immunisation. Reports of congenital rubella syndrome in the UK have significantly reduced since the introduction of the two dose MMR schedule, but a reduction in the number of children being given MMR because of health scares in the media might lead to a resurgence of the problem for susceptible individuals in the future.

Influenza immunisation

Influenza vaccine is produced each year with the three strains of virus likely to be circulating during the winter season. Annual injections of 0.5 ml SC or IM are required. Patients at particular risk who should be targeted include:

- Patients with medical conditions likely to be exacerbated by influenza: diabetes, asthma, chronic respiratory, heart or renal disease
- Immunosuppressed patients
- Residents in institutions where a rapid spread of infection would be likely to occur
- All patients aged over 65 years.

Front line healthcare workers are also offered immunisation by occupational health services[15].

Preparation for the immunisation programme should be made early. Vaccines can be bought in bulk from the manufacturer, if suitable storage is available. A profit for the practice can be made this way. Alternatively, individual patients are issued with a prescription for the vaccine, which they get from the chemist and return for the injection. Patients at risk can be identified from disease and age/sex registers. Special flu jab clinics may be set up and invitations sent out. The best time to start the programme is early October. In this way the bulk of the injections will be completed before the end of the year to protect patients early in the following year when influenza epidemics are most likely. Patients who are not in the risk categories or who do not have a valid need for immunisation should be discouraged from having flu injections in case there is insufficient vaccine available for those at true risk.

Contraindications

Contraindications to influenza vaccine include:

- Any febrile illness (postpone injection until recovered)
- Severe adverse reaction to a previous dose
- Hypersensitivity to egg (previous anaphylactic reaction)
- Pregnancy.

Adverse reactions are usually mild. Soreness may occur at the injection site. Fever, malaise or myalgia may occur a few hours after immunisation and last up to two days. Very rarely there might be an allergic reaction if the patient is hypersensitive to egg protein, because the virus is cultured in eggs to produce the vaccine. Many patients refuse the flu vaccine because they believe it gives them the flu. Discussion with the patient about the influenza vaccine; the type of vaccine, the efficacy of the vaccine and the benefits it provides will give patients a more informed choice. Flu vaccine is inactivated so cannot cause flu in recipients or their contacts.

Pneumococcal immunisation

An encapsulated strain of *Streptococcus pneumoniae* can cause pneumonia, bacteraemia or meningitis. Susceptible patients who should be offered immunisation include people with:

- Chronic lung, heart, liver or renal conditions
- Disorders of immunity through disease or treatment
- Diabetes mellitus
- Disease of spleen or splenectomy
- Homozygous sickle cell disease.

A single dose of 23-valent pneumococcal vaccine 0.5 ml SC or IM is required. It may be given at the same time as a flu jab, but at a different injection site.

At present there are no firm guidelines on re-vaccinating with pneumococcal immunisation. However, the British Committee for Standards in Haematology Guideline advises re-immunisation in asplenic patients to be five-yearly but other particular circumstances may be made on antibody levels, which in patients with sickle cell anaemia and lymphoproliferative disorders may decline more rapidly[16]. Adverse reactions include possible mild soreness at injection site and slight fever.

Possible future developments

A 7-valent conjugated pneumococcal vaccine Prevenar has been licensed in the UK. This license applies from the age of six months to two years (those previously not covered by the 23-valent pneumococcal vaccine). Manufacturers' guidelines recommend its use within the childhood primary immunisation schedule and at 12–15 months of age. The Joint Committee on Vaccines and Immunisations (JCVI) has not yet issued guidelines on the use of Prevenar.

Hepatitis B

This highly infectious virus is spread by blood contact through contaminated sharps or needles, sexual intercourse, mother to child at birth, or a bite from an infected person.

Active immunisation

Immunisation is recommended for people at particular risk:

- Healthcare personnel
- Patient contacts from haemodialysis, haematology or oncology departments
- Plasma fraction workers
- Drug abusers
- Patients at increased risk due to sexual activities, including some homosexual men
- Travellers going to reside in areas where hepatitis B is endemic
- Close contacts with patients with hepatitis B or healthy carriers of the virus.

The recombinant hepatitis B vaccine is prepared from yeast cells. Three intramuscular doses of 1 ml are required for adults at birth, one and six months. (0.5 ml for children 0–12 years). An accelerated schedule may be used (see Green Book). Injection should be into the deltoid muscle instead of the buttock. (The antero-lateral thigh should be used for infants.) Patients with bleeding disorders, when an intramuscular injection could cause bleeding into the muscle, may be given subcutaneous injection at the discretion of the GP. A higher dose vaccine (40 mcg) is available for patients with renal failure who are undergoing dialysis.

Antibody levels should be checked about 2–4 months after the completion of the primary course. Further doses are sometimes required to achieve initial immunity levels of 100 iu/ml. One reinforcing dose five years after the successful primary course is recommended, without serology testing. Adverse reactions include redness and soreness at the injection site. More rarely there is fever, rash, flu-like symptoms, arthralgia and/or abnormal liver function tests.

Hepatitis A

Protection against hepatitis A is usually required for travellers. However, now that active immunisation is possible it should be considered for occupational groups at particular risk, for example, sewerage workers. Carers and residents in institutions, where outbreaks of hepatitis A are likely, may also be considered for immunisation. Two injections are required for lasting immunity, given intramuscularly into the deltoid muscle; the second dose administered 6–12 months after the first. Gay men may benefit from a hepatitis A and B combined vaccine (Twinrix,) as there is a greater risk of acquiring both diseases in this group. Human normal immunoglobulin (HBIG) is no longer used for short-term travel but may still be used in certain outbreak situations.

Conclusion

The input by health professionals is greatest in the early years of an individual's life. Checks and charts seem to rule. It is important that these continue to enable a secure environment for our children. Events such as the Victoria Climbié case highlight the importance for professionals to work within a multidisciplinary team with good communication. It is important for health professionals to understand their roles and responsibilities when working with children and adequate training is required.

Achieving a high uptake of immunisation makes a worthwhile contribution to the health of the population. Practice nurses provide a vaccination service, but time also needs to be made available when planning appointments, to help educate the public about transmission of infectious diseases. It is important that health professionals are kept up to date with vaccines and vaccine policy. Aitkin, Lunt *et al.* found that further education on vaccination was not often felt necessary, as nurses were dealing with these on a daily basis[17].

With media publicity on MMR, health professionals have realised that they are not able to effectively answer the questions asked by members of the public or, indeed, do not have the knowledge to understand the controversy. With the success of the national vaccination programme, many parents will not have seen first hand the effects of the diseases that have now largely been prevented.

The introduction of meningitis C in recent times has shown the effectiveness of the immunisation programme, and it is when the incidence of disease is low, that vaccine safety becomes an issue. Due to public anxiety about the safety and efficacy of pertussis vaccine, uptake rate fell to 30% in 1975. Then, health professionals were not confident with the evidence presented and felt that by offering a choice (DTP or DT) parents were choosing the safest option for their child. Unfortunately this resulted in several major epidemics with over 100 000 notified cases.

Suggestions for reflection on practice

- Should one individual's rights be allowed to compromise another person's individual rights?

Further reading

Kassanios, G. (2001) *Immunisation Childhood and Travel Health*, 4th edn. Blackwell Science, Oxford.

World Health Organisation (1996) WHO-VHPB Communicable Disease Series No 1. *Prevention and Control of Hepatitis B in the Community*. World Health Organization, Geneva.

References

1. Luker, K. & Orr, J. (eds) (1992) *Health Visiting: Towards Community Health Nursing*. Blackwell Science, Oxford.
2. Hertfordshire (East and North Hertfordshire Health Authority and West Hertfordshire Health Authority) (2000) *Pre-School Child Health Surveillance and Health Promotion. A manual for Hertfordshire*, 2nd edn. Watford Printers, Watford.
3. Glazener, C., Ramsay, C., Campbell, M., *et al.* (1999) Neonatal examination and screening trial (NEST): a randomised, controlled, switchback trial of alternative policies for low risk infants. *British Medical Journal*, **318**, 627–32.
4. Baron-Cohen, S., Allen, J. & Gillberg, C. (1992) Can autism be detected at 18 months? The needle, the haystack, and the CHAT. *British Journal of Psychiatry*, **161**, 839–43.
5. White, A. (2001) The drive to reduce the number of teenage pregnancies. *Community Outlook*, June, 11.
6. Department of Health (1999) *Working Together to Safeguard Children*. HMSO, London.
7. Department of Health (2001) *Consent – What you have a right to expect. A guide for children and young people*. Department of Health, London. *www.doh.open.gov.uk/consent*
8. Department of Health (1996) *Immunisation against Infectious Disease*. HMSO, London.
9. Department of Health (2000) *Health Service Circular* HSC 2000/026 Patient Group Directions (England only).
10. Department of Health (1990) *A Guide to Consent for Treatment*, HC 90. Department of Health, London.
11. Shire Hall Communications (2001) *UK Guidance on Best Practice in Vaccine Administration*. Shire Hall Communications, London.
12. Miller, E. (1999) Overview of recent clinical trials of acellular pertussis vaccines. *Biologicals*, **27** (2), 79–86.
13. Department of Health CMO, CNO and CPhO Letter (2001) *Pre-school acellular pertussis booster*. PL/CMO2001/5, PL/CNO/2001/7, PL/CPHO/20001/5, Department of Health, London.

14. Diggle, L. & Deeks, J. (2000) Routine primary immunisation using a longer needle resulted in fewer local reactions in infants. *British Medical Journal*, **321**, 931–933.

15. Department of Health (2001) *New Service Standards for 2001/02* (2001/02 SERVICE STANDARDS) – Reflecting the true patient experience. *www.doh.gov.uk/winter/issues*

16. Davies, J.M. (2001) The prevention and treatment of infection in patients with an absent or dysfunctional spleen: updated guideline. *British Medical Journal*, 2 June.

17. Atkin, K., Lunt, N., Parker, G. & Hirst, M. (1993) *Nurses Count: A National Census of Practice Nurses*. Social Policy Research Unit, York.

Useful addresses and web sites

Public Health Laboratory Services
Communicable Disease Surveillance Centre, 61 Colindale Avenue, London NW9 5HT
Telephone: 020 8200 6868.

Web sites

www.phls.org.uk Public Health Laboratory Service.
www.immunisation.org.com Health Promotion England.
www.nct-online.org National Childbirth Trust.
www.doh.gov.uk Department of Health.

Chapter 11
Travel Health

With travellers becoming increasingly adventurous and virtually no country inaccessible, travel health advisers should remember that their pre-travel consultations should concentrate mainly on the advice they give and how important it is to follow good guidelines on subjects such as food hygiene and bite prevention. Sensible behaviour is the key to good health, and vaccination and preventative medicine are simply added safeguards.

Research has shown that cardiovascular disease was the largest cause of death in (Scottish) travellers abroad (69% of deaths), with 21% caused by accidents and injuries and only 4% of deaths caused by infection[1]. Of all the problems occurring, the majority were associated with pre-existing conditions which would have been identifiable before travel. Therefore, with the frequency of travel to exotic destinations rising in the older age-group, it is wise for the adviser to take a careful history and to tailor his/her advice and preventive measures to individual patients. Many practice nurses have assumed the responsibility for travel health, which by its complexity, calls for high standards of care. The nurse should have adequate education and knowledge about travel health, access to suitable reference material, and work to appropriate guidelines.

Nurse education

There are many opportunities to access study days, including those run by local trusts, travel centres and vaccine producers. More specialised, accredited training is also available through postgraduate study. These include:

- Short courses in travel health run by Staffordshire University, Queen Margaret College, Edinburgh and the London School of Hygiene and Tropical Medicine
- Diplomas in travel medicine available through Glasgow University and the Royal Free Hospital School of Medicine, London
- Distance learning can be undertaken with the Magister Learning Unit in Travel Health

- Combined distance learning and taught sessions with the Lancaster University Travel Medicine Course.

Sources of advice

The following provide advice:

- *Immunisation against Infectious Diseases*[2] (the Green Book) and *International Travel and Health*[3] (the Yellow Book) should be standard reference books
- A computerised system gives regular updates via a modern link to the Medical Advisory Services for Travellers Abroad (MASTA) or TRAVAX run by the Scottish Centre for Infection and Environmental Health
- Information on disease risks and immunisation is published in *Pulse, MIMS* and other journals
- Telephone information services run by vaccine companies such as Aventis Pasteur MSD, provide information about health risks and injections
- There are many textbooks providing information on all aspects of travel health. For example *Travel Medicine and Migrant Health*[4], and *Immunisation Childhood and Travel Health*[5].
- The booklet *Health Advice for Travellers* is available from the Department of Health and local health promotion departments (the booklet has regular updates so, in order to have the most up-to-date information for patients, excess ordering should be avoided)
- *The Rough Guide to Travel Health* provides sensible advice for all travellers as well as information on more exotic travel problems[6].

It is helpful if patients fill in a form outlining their travel plans and immunisation status, so that advice can be tailored to their needs. Samples of these could be on the practice computer system, or be obtained from the PCT or from vaccine companies. Specialist help can be needed with complicated itineraries. MASTA will provide written health briefs for individual patients, so it is useful to keep a stock of information cards giving the contact number.

Advice for travellers

Food and water

Diarrhoea is the most common problem for travellers. Detailed advice on hand washing and food and water safety may prevent a journey from becoming a disaster. Bacteria multiply more quickly in hot climates so extra special care is needed where hygiene standards are suspect.

Advice	Rationale
Eat freshly prepared and cooked hot food	Before bacterial growth can occur in cooked food and after any bacteria have been destroyed by heat
Avoid salads and choose raw fruits and vegetables that can be peeled	Human excreta may be used as fertiliser or unsafe water may be used to wash the food
Avoid shellfish	Their feeding method concentrates micro-organisms from their environment within their bodies
Boil or avoid unpasteurised milk	Risk of tuberculosis or brucellosis
Avoid ice creams, especially those in multi-portion containers	Ingredients could be hazardous, especially if ice cream has melted and been refrozen
Avoid raw meat and fish	Worm infestation risk
Boil or sterilise unsafe water or used bottled water	Water could be contaminated with human or animal excreta
Check the seal is unbroken on any bottled water purchased	To ensure that the bottle has not been refilled with tap water
Avoid ice cubes in drinks and use safe water for cleaning teeth	Even small amounts of unsafe water could be hazardous
Check that recreational water is safe	Swimming pools may be contaminated if not well-maintained; there is a risk of bilharzia in some fresh-water areas; sea water may have sewage contamination

Diarrhoea advice

If diarrhoea does occur most cases will resolve within two to three days. Whatever the cause, dehydration is the major complication, so fluid replacement is essential. Mildly affected healthy adults may only need plenty of non-alcoholic drinks, including fruit juices and soups, but in all other cases, rehydration fluid should be used – either a solution made from a commercially produced sachet or four heaped teaspoonfuls of sugar or honey and one level teaspoonful of salt in one litre of safe water. One glass should be drunk after each motion. Small, regular amounts should be continued even if vomiting occurs. Starvation is not recommended. Breastfeeding for infants should also be continued. Medical help should be obtained for very young children, elderly or frail people, those with other medical conditions like diabetes, or if diarrhoea contains blood or the patient becomes more ill.

Anti-diarrhoea medication may be needed by adults, e.g. on long bus journeys or on business trips. Anti-diarrhoea drugs are not recommended for children or for patients with bloody diarrhoea[7]. A short course of antibiotics can reduce the severity and duration of travellers' diarrhoea[8]. The decision on which patients should carry self-treatment will depend on the practice policy; private prescriptions should be issued for any medication prescribed for this purpose. Diarrhoea can make the contraceptive pill ineffective so patients should be advised to carry alternative methods of contraception.

Malaria

Female anopheline mosquitoes transmit the parasites that cause malaria in their saliva. Protection against bites is often more important than drug prophylaxis because drug resistance is becoming such a serious problem. Of the four species of malaria parasites, *Plasmodium falciparum* is the most serious, causing death in about 1% of travellers infected. Up-to-date information on anti-malarial drugs is supplied by the Malaria Reference Laboratory. Travellers at risk on long trips to remote places should also have drugs and information for treating malaria, in case infection does occur. People who previously have lived in a malarious area must be warned of their particular risk when returning, as they may have lost their previous immunity but fail to take adequate precautions against mosquito bites. Advice on malaria should cover the following points:

- Personal protection: since mosquitoes feed mainly after dusk and at dawn, keep arms, legs and feet covered after sunset and avoid perfume and dark clothing.

- Use insect repellents containing diethyl tolumide (DEET), or similar chemicals, to deter biting and try to obtain preparations with the highest DEET content available (these may be applied to the skin with caution, or clothes can be impregnated with DEET or permethrin for a more lasting effect; impregnated wrist and ankle bands may also be helpful).

- Protection at night: if using air conditioning, make sure that windows and doors are closed properly and use an insecticide spray if necessary.

- If mosquitoes are able to enter at night use a mosquito net. Make sure it has no holes or tears and tuck it properly under the mattress, preferably before dusk. Ensure that the net is large enough to allow plenty of space between the sleeper and the net because if their body is in contact with the net the mosquitoes can still attack through it! Nets impregnated with permethrin will kill or repel mosquitoes, so are more effective.

- Pyrethroid mosquito coils or electrically operated vaporisers may also be of use, providing they last until daybreak. Electricity supplies are often unreliable.

- Malaria can develop whilst travelling and, in some instances, up to a year after it. If travellers experience flu-like symptoms and fever, especially if associated with rigors, they should seek medical help as soon as possible. If they have already returned home they should inform the doctor that they have been to a malarious area.

- Early treatment of malaria can prevent a fatal outcome[9].

The potential risk of malaria needs to be established and the appropriate prophylaxis advised. Charts are published monthly in *Pulse*, *MIMS* and other journals, giving the recommended anti-malarial regimes. To ensure the parity of care, all team members should use the same information source, as there can be differences. Chloroquine and proguanil can be purchased in a pharmacy. A private prescription is required for mefloquine, doxycycline, Malarone and Maloprim.

No anti-malarial tablets are 100% effective, and none will prevent infection occurring. Their main effect, with the exception of Malarone, is to impede the four-week life cycle of the parasite after the liver stage. Hence the need to continue taking most tablets for at least four weeks after leaving the risk area and to seek medical advice if symptoms occur. All the tablets can cause nausea and gastric disturbance. All tablets should be taken with food and swallowed whole with plenty of water. The inconvenience of side effects can be minimised by evening dosing.

Unless otherwise stated, tablets should be started one week before arrival, to ensure an adequate level of drug in the bloodstream, taken continuously throughout stay and for four weeks after leaving the malarious area. Tablets should be taken as prescribed. Missing doses can be as bad as taking no tablets at all. Patients should be warned about possible side effects (see *BNF*).

Malaria prophylaxis

Drug	Contraindications/cautions	Advice
Proguanil (Paludrine) Daily dose	Caution in renal impairment May potentiate the effect of warfarin Folate supplements needed in pregnancy	Seek specialist advice Blood test pre- and post-travel to stabilise the dose 5 mg, daily recommended dose
Chloroquine (Avloclor, Nivaquine) Weekly dose	Contraindicated with epilepsy May aggravate psoriasis Caution with liver and renal impairment	Consider doxycycline as an alternative Seek specialist advice

(Continued)

Drug (continued)	Contraindications/cautions (continued)	Advice (continued)
Mefloquine (Lariam) Daily dose Commence tablets 2.5–3 weeks before departure to allow time to change to another drug if side effects occur	Contraindicated if: – history of mental illness – convulsions or epilepsy – pregnant, breast-feeding, or planning a pregnancy within three months of trip – severe liver, heart, kidney disease Vivid dreams and dizziness can occur	Use alternative anti-malarial Ensure adequate supplies of contraceptives Get medical advice Caution if driving
Doxycycline (Vibramycin) Daily dose Commence two days prior to arrival in malarious area	Contraindicated in: – pregnancy and lactation – children Caution with liver disease Can cause oesophagitis Can cause sun sensitivity	Use alternative drug or seek specialist advice Take after food with plenty of water, while standing or sitting straight Cover up and use high factor suncream
Atovaquone with proguanil (Malarone) Daily dose Commence 24–48 hours prior to arrival and continue until seven days after leaving the malarious area	Licensed for trips up to 28 days, i.e. up to 37 tablets. The time license may be extended in the future	The tablets are expensive Patients should be aware of the cost before the prescription is written
Pyrimethamine and dapsone (Maloprim) Weekly dose	Not suitable for children under five years	Folate supplements needed in pregnancy and deficiency states[10]

All anti-malarial drugs can have unwanted side effects. Patients should be advised to read the leaflet supplied with the tablets and know what problems could occur.

Sun exposure

Patients should be warned about the risks of exposure to too much sun. Long-term exposure can cause skin cancer; especially as the ozone layer which filters out dangerous ultraviolet radiation is being destroyed. Sunburn may ruin a holiday and in extreme cases, could be fatal. Falling asleep in the sun is a big danger and is often caused by excessive alcohol intake. Generally speaking, the fairer the skin, the greater the risk of burning. Children need special vigilance and protection from the sun.

Sensible precautions for sunbathers should include gradual acclimatisation (beginning with only ten to fifteen minutes a day in the morning or mid-afternoon) and the regular application of sunscreens with a minimum of SPF 15. Reapplication will be needed after swimming or showering. Water, sand and snow will all increase the reflection of ultraviolet, so extra care is needed to protect skin on beaches, ski-slopes or when taking part in water sports. A moisturising cream should be applied after exposure to the sun and regular drinks are needed to replace fluid loss. Alcohol causes dehydration and should, therefore, be limited. If urine is dark and concentrated then more fluids are needed. Salt lost in sweat will also need replacing, either in the diet, or in excessive sweating, by also adding half a level teaspoonful of salt per litre of liquid for drinking. Severe sunburn will need medical treatment.

Heatstroke

Heatstroke may happen without direct exposure to the sun. Impairment of the heat-regulating system causes a dangerous rise in body temperature as sweating diminishes. Death can occur within a few hours if not treated. Immediate cooling by evaporation is needed, using wet sheets or towels on the skin, and fanning. Rehydration with cool drinks is also essential, and emergency medical treatment should be obtained. Patients should be warned of the contributing factors to heatstroke, especially for anyone with a skin condition that impairs sweating. These include:

- Continuous heat stress
- Lack of fitness, obesity
- Alcohol excess
- Strenuous exercise
- Too much or unsuitable clothing
- Some drugs, including cold remedies and diuretics[11].

Blood-borne viruses and sexually transmitted diseases

The holiday atmosphere and alcohol may combine to remove inhibitions but may also result in unwanted souvenirs. Casual sexual encounters lead to the spread of sexually transmitted diseases (including blood-borne viruses). The prostitutes in many countries could be infected and patients should be warned of the serious risks. If used correctly, condoms provide a degree of protection, but they should be stored in a cool place away from direct sunlight and particular care is needed to prevent their being damaged in transit. The quality of condoms available in countries outside the UK may not be as high, so travellers, both male and female, should be encouraged to take a supply with them.

Tattooing, acupuncture, and body piercing should be avoided. Emergency medical or dental treatment may expose travellers to risk in countries where the reuse of equipment is likely. Sterile emergency packs containing, syringes, needles, sutures and blood transfusion needles can be purchased for a reasonable price but blood transfusion and dental work should be avoided if at all possible in high risk countries. Travellers should be advised to have sufficient health insurance to be repatriated in an emergency.

Accidents

Some patients worry about catching exotic diseases and request a plethora of immunisations, whereas in reality, they are probably far more at risk of accidental injury or even death. Alcohol excess leading to risk-taking, dangerous transport and driving conditions, or drowning are just some of the hazards travellers should consider seriously. The risks of violence to travellers, particularly in countries with civil unrest, are a major concern. Nurses can only advise patients to do their homework and be aware of any potential problems. The choice of where to travel lies with the patient. Every attempt should be made to obey the laws of the country being visited.

High altitude

The reduced atmospheric pressure at high altitudes means that less oxygen is available to the tissues. The body adapts by deeper respirations and a faster heart rate, but time for acclimatisation is necessary and fatalities do occur. Patients planning journeys to high altitudes (over 2400 m) should seek medical advice; especially if they have respiratory or cardiac conditions, or sickle cell anaemia.

Air travel

Flying at high altitude, despite cabin pressurisation, may also cause problems of hypoxia for some people, particularly those who smoke heavily. The ears are likely to be affected by changes in air pressure, and severe discomfort may be caused if congestion blocks the Eustachian tubes. Patients with medical problems should ask a doctor to check their fitness to fly.

The venous return can be slowed when sitting in a cramped seat for long periods and can cause a deep vein thrombosis (DVT). The effects of air travel on health were the subject of an enquiry by a Select Committee of the House of Lords. Among the recommendations on seating, ventilation and air quality, was advice that health professionals stop using the term *economy class syndrome* because first-class and business passengers or people using other forms of long-distance transport could be equally vulnerable. *Travellers' thrombosis* was thought to be a more appropriate term[12]. While more research has yet to be undertaken, recent publicity around the risk of DVT has led to several preventative recommendations. These include leg and stretching exercises, standing up and drinking plenty of water, but reducing alcohol intake. For travellers at risk from DVT, e.g. those undergoing hormone treatments, with malignancy and who have had any recent major surgery, additional measures should be discussed with the GP. These measures may include graduated compression hosiery, aspirin or low dose heparin[13].

Travel in pregnancy

Always ask 'Is your journey really necessary?' Pregnant women should be advised not to travel to remote areas, but if such travel is essential, then between 18 and 24 weeks gestation are considered to be the most suitable times[14]. Air travel in normal pregnancy is generally considered safe up to 35 weeks, but women should check with their particular airline. There is a greater risk of thromboembolic disease in pregnancy. A doctor's letter may be required and adequate health insurance, which covers pregnancy, is essential.

Immunisation should be avoided in pregnancy, except when the risk from the disease outweighs the risk from the vaccine. All risks should be discussed with the woman and any immunisation must be prescribed by the GP. Pregnant women are more likely to be seriously affected by malaria, which can induce premature delivery or spontaneous abortion[14]. Proguanil and chloroquine at normal doses can be used with 5 mg folic acid tablets taken daily. Specialist advice should be sought for pregnant travellers going to chloroquine-resistant areas.

Travel with children

Special care is needed when travelling with young children. Dehydration and sun exposure should be avoided. Skincare is important, as prickly heat and nappy rash are more common in hot climates[15]. All routine childhood immunisations should be up to date. BCG and hepatitis B can be given at birth and an accelerated course of hep. B given if necessary, with a booster dose 12 months later. Travel vaccinations are not normally given to children aged under one year and typhoid vaccine is less effective before 18 months of age. Exposure to hepatitis A in childhood, whilst not causing severe symptoms in most children, will confer life-long immunity. Immunisation would be mainly as a public health measure aimed at the prevention of spread of the disease. Immunisation is recommended for children of immigrant parents, born in western Europe, before visiting countries where hepatitis A is endemic[16].

Travel for patients with respiratory diseases

Travellers with pre-existing respiratory problems will find they are more at risk of contracting respiratory illnesses whilst abroad. A respiratory health check is advisable before departure to ensure that the patient is fit to travel and knows what to do if unwell.

Care should be taken to:

- Carry sufficient inhalers for the trip – some in hand luggage and some in main luggage
- Be aware of the signs of deterioration of their condition and know when to commence emergency treatment
- Have a standby course of emergency medication
- Carry a large spacer device and MDI (metered dose inhaler) of a reliever, for medical emergencies
- Carry a doctor's letter to outline current treatment
- Plan trip to avoid known trigger factors
- Ensure health insurance is adequate
- Consider vaccination against pneumonia and influenza.

Travel for patients with diabetes

Patients with diabetes should obtain advice before long journeys, especially if crossing time zones. These points should be considered:

- Ensure you have sufficient medication etc. for the entire trip.
- Carry emergency carbohydrates in the hand luggage (food may not be allowed on aircraft since foot and mouth disease precautions were instituted: glucose tablets or Lucozade are recommended by Diabetes UK instead).
- Carry all the insulin in the hand luggage (in case baggage gets mislaid, and because the insulin could freeze in the hold if travelling by air). Use an insulated bag to keep the insulin cool. Carry blood monitoring kit in hand luggage. Airlines have imposed stringent rules about hand luggage in response to international terrorism and it would be sensible to have a doctor's letter. It would also be wise to contact the airline in advance[17]. Dietary requirements should also be explained.
- Take medication, if needed, to prevent travel sickness.
- Follow the normal sickness advice if vomiting or diarrhoea occur (see Appendix 3).
- Make sure the travel insurance is adequate, and that the insurer knows about the diabetes. Diabetes UK will advise patients.
- Carry E111 form if travelling within the European Union.

Immunisation for travellers

Practice nurses usually work out the schedules and administer immunisations for travellers under patient group directions (PGD). Each nurse should maintain an up-to-date, signed PGD and also have clear guidelines as to when a doctor should be consulted regarding travel health consultations. Many surgeries now purchase the vaccines and claim reimbursement and dispensing fees. The storage of vaccines needs special care and temperature control (see Chapter 4).

Immunisation serves two purposes: to prevent the spread of diseases and to protect the individual from infection. Proof of immunisation may be mandatory in some countries and entry can be denied without a valid certificate of immunisation. Yellow fever is the only disease for which an International Certificate of Immunisation may still be required. Cholera certificates are still demanded in some countries, although immunisation is no longer recommended by the World Health Organisation. Travellers to the Hajj in Saudi Arabia require proof of meningitis immunisation.

Individual schedules of immunisation will depend on:

- The injections previously received
- The length and type of journey
- The time available before departure.

Accelerated schedules are possible, but it is best to start 6–8 weeks before departure (14 weeks if a full course of tetanus and/or polio is needed). Some diseases are seasonal, so up-to-date information is necessary. The travel charts in *Pulse, MIMS* etc. are suitable for straightforward trips. The telephone information services and MASTA will advise on more complicated journeys, or the practice may have computer access to a database. The Green Book gives essential information about all the vaccines, doses, contraindications and side effects.

The safeguards and emergency procedures should be specified in the patient group directions. All the vaccines administered and specific advice given must be recorded accurately in the patients' records. Computer records of immunisation save time when planning future schedules and are valuable for administration and audit purposes also. Item of service fees may be claimed for most immunisations but this is a complicated situation, which will need clarification locally. Fees for temporary residents cannot be claimed as well as item of service fees if only immunisations are given, but both are allowed if travel health or other medical advice is given as well.

Contraindications to immunisation

A check list helps to ensure that no essential questions are omitted:

Questions	Rationale
Are you well today? (if the answer is 'no', check what the problem is)	Postpone immunisation if acute or febrile illness
Are you taking steroids or have you any condition which affects your immune system?	Live viruses should not be given to immunosuppressed patients
Is there any chance that you might be pregnant? (female patients)	Vaccines should not be administered unless risk of disease outweighs possible risk to the fetus; consult the GP

(Continued)

Questions (continued)	Rationale (continued)
Have you reacted badly to any previous vaccine?	Medical advice needed before the vaccine is given
Are you allergic to eggs?	Previous anaphylactic reaction to eggs may contraindicate vaccines such as yellow fever made from viruses cultured in eggs

The manufacturers' instructions for administration and contraindications to immunisation must always be observed.

Tetanus

The risk of tetanus occurs throughout the world. Spores of the bacillus are found in the soil and can thus be transmitted to humans through wounds. The faeces of domestic animals may also contain the spores. A primary course or booster is recommended for anyone not already protected (see Chapter 10).

Poliomyelitis

Polio is still prevalent in many developing countries. A primary course or booster is recommended for anyone, who is not fully immunised, planning to travel outside northern Europe, Australia, New Zealand or the Americas (see Chapter 10). There are also exceptions for short-term travellers to some other countries where the wild poliomyelitis virus has been eradicated.

Typhoid

Typhoid fever is a *Salmonella* infection transmitted by food or water contaminated by the faeces either of a person suffering from the disease, or from a chronic carrier who has recovered from the disease but still excretes the bacterium. The infection causes a systemic disease, which can be fatal if untreated. The food and drink precautions given above are important but immunisation is also recommended for many areas.

- Vi capsular polysaccharide vaccine: one dose gives protection for 3 years.
- Attenuated live oral vaccine is a live oral vaccine consisting of three capsules; one to be taken on alternate days. Three capsules give protection for three years, but the instructions for storing the capsules and timing the doses must be followed. It is not recommended for children under six years old.

Hepatitis A

Hepatitis A is a viral infection caused by faecal contamination of food and water. The disease is usually mild in young children and may not be recognised but they can still transmit the infection. Vaccines for active immunisation have been available for many years. Two doses give protection for up to ten years. Passive immunisation with immunoglobulin is no longer recommended because of the risk of transmitting infection from the donor. Blood can be taken beforehand to test for hepatitis A antibodies, if previous infection is thought likely to have occurred. Laboratories in some areas may charge a private fee for such tests.

Hepatitis B

Immunisation against the hepatitis B virus is not routinely recommended for short-term travel but it may be offered to people planning to spend long periods abroad and to travellers likely to be at special risk through their work or lifestyle. Patients should know that hepatitis B is spread through contact with blood and other body fluids and the measures to take to avoid that contact.

Newer vaccines are available which combine hepatitis A and typhoid vaccines and hepatitis A and B vaccines. These may be useful for reducing the number of injections for patients who are afraid of needles or when time is limited before departure. Combined vaccines may not attract the same item of service fees, so this should be checked locally. Immunisation against hepatitis A will require a separate booster if the first dose is combined with typhoid vaccine.

Yellow fever

Yellow fever is a viral infection transmitted by mosquito bites in tropical Africa and South America. The incubation period is 3–6 days. Immunisation is given only at designated centres, but with the increase in foreign travel, many practices have now been accepted as yellow fever centres by the Department of Health. At times when only unlicensed vaccine is available, the GP must decide if it is to be offered and must prescribe the vaccine for individual patients. Unlicensed vaccine cannot be given under a PGD. An International Certificate of Immunisation against Yellow Fever is issued after immunisation and becomes valid ten days after immunisation. One dose conveys immunity for ten years, so patients should be advised to take care of their certificates during that time. A private fee can be charged because the vaccine has to be purchased and is not reimbursable. Patients from other surgeries may be seen privately for yellow fever immunisation. Suitable records must be kept.

Meningococcal meningitis

Meningococcal meningitis usually occurs in epidemics. It is a bacterial infection spread by droplets, so is most common in areas where people are crowded together. Some visitors to the 'meningitis belt of Africa', northern India, and the lowlands of Nepal during the dry seasons could be at risk of meningitis. One dose of meningitis A and C vaccine provides immunity for three to five years for adults and children over two months of age. A newer meningitis vaccine against A, C, W and Y strains is available for travellers to areas where these types of the disease are endemic. Visitors to the Hajj in Mecca should be given this vaccine; they will be denied entry to Saudi Arabia without a certificate of meningitis immunisation. The vaccine must have been given not more than three years before, or less than ten days previously, for the certificate to be valid.

Rabies

Rabies is a viral infection, usually transmitted by the bite or saliva of an infected animal. Pre-exposure immunisation may be offered to travellers to remote areas where they may be more than 24 hours journey time away from a hospital. A course of three injections provides some protection for up to three years. The vaccine is usually prescribed on a private prescription. Post-exposure treatment is still needed if bitten. A patient who is scratched or bitten by an animal which could have rabies should also be advised:

* To cleanse the wound thoroughly with soap and water
* To get the name and address of the animal's owner (if known), so the animal can be observed for signs of rabies
* To get advice from a local doctor about the risk of rabies in that area.

Patients who need rabies immunisation may also need to carry tablets for the self-treatment of malaria if they are likely to be at risk in remote areas, without immediate access to medical facilities.

Japanese B encephalitis

Japanese B encephalitis is a viral disease spread by mosquitoes, most commonly found in rural areas of Asian countries during the monsoon season, where there are concentrations of pigs and birds near rice fields. The prevention of mosquito bites is the best preventive measure. An inactivated vaccine is available on a named-patient basis only on a private prescription. Severe allergic reactions can occur after immunisation and delayed reactions are possible. The need for the vaccine must be weighed against possible risks of the disease, with further advice being sought if necessary.

Tick-borne encephalitis

Tick-borne encephalitis is caused by a virus transmitted by the bite of an infected animal tick; mainly during the spring and summer. Ticks are picked up from the undergrowth in warm, forested areas of Europe and Scandinavia. Hikers and campers are most at risk. People planning trips to those areas should be advised not to walk with bare legs and to use an insect repellent. A killed vaccine is available on a named-patient basis. A full course to last three years requires three injections. Two injections give protection for one year.

Suggestions for reflection on practice

How effective is your travel health service?

- Are appointment times long enough to provide comprehensive advice?
- Are your knowledge and reference materials up to date?

References

1. Paixio, M., Dewar, R., Cossar, J. *et al.* (1991) What do Scots die of when abroad? *Scottish Medical Journal*, **36**, 114–16.
2. Department of Health (1996) *Immunisation against Infectious Disease*. HMSO, London.
3. World Health Organisation (2001) *International Travel and Health – Vaccination requirements and Health Advice*. HMSO, London.
4. Lockie, C., Walker, E., Calvert, L., Cossar, J., Knill-Jones, R. & Raeside, F. (eds) (2000) *Travel Medicine and Migrant Health*. Churchill Livingstone, Edinburgh.
5. Kassianos, G. (2001) *Immunisation, Childhood and Travel Health*. Blackwell Science, Oxford.
6. Jones, N. (2001) *The Rough Guide to Travel Health*. Rough Guides, London.
7. Farthing, M. (1998) Travellers' diarrhoea: mechanisms, manifestations and management. *Medicine*, 33–9.
8. Caeiro, J. & Dupont, H. (1998) Management of travellers' diarrhoea. *Drugs*, **56**, 73–81.
9. Author not known (1997) *The ABC of Healthy Travel*. BMJ Publishing Group, Cambridge.
10. Kassianos, G. (2001) *Immunisation, Childhood and Travel Health*, pp. 375–82. Blackwell Science, Oxford.
11. Adam, J. (1992) In: *Travellers' Health – How to stay healthy abroad*, R. Dawood (ed.) pp. 237–8. Oxford University Press, Oxford.
12. House of Lords, Select Committee on Science and Technology (2000) *Air Travel and Health*. HMSO, London.
13. Geroulakos, G. (2001) The risk of venous thromboembolism from air travel. *British Medical Journal*, **322**, 188.
14. Simpson, M. (2000) Women and child travellers. In: *Travel Medicine and Migrant Health* (eds C. Lockie, E. Walker, L. Calvert, J. Cossar, R. Knill-Jones & F. Raeside). Churchill Livingstone, Edinburgh.
15. Ganley, Y. (1996) *Handbook of Travel Medicine*. Science Press, London.
16. Kassianos, G. (2001) *Immunisation, Childhood and Travel Health*, p. 150, Blackwell Science, Oxford.
17. Diabetes UK (2001) *Air travel and insulin. www.diabetes.org.uk/news/sept01/airtravel.* (accessed 3/10/01).

Useful addresses and web sites

Aventis Pasteur MSD Vaccine Information Service
Telephone: 07000 766 73847

Medical Advisory Service for Travellers Abroad (MASTA)
Keppel Street, London WC1E 7HT
Telephone Travellers Healthline: 09068 224 100

PHLS Malaria Reference Laboratory
London School of Hygiene and Tropical Medicine
Keppel Street, London WC1E 7HT
Telephone: 0207 636 3924 (for advice for health professionals)
Premium line telephone: 09065 508 908 (advice line for the general public)
Web site: *www.lsthm.ac.uk/itd/units/pmbbu/malaria/malariaref*

Scottish Centre for Infection and Environmental Health
Clifton House, Clifton Place, Glasgow G3 7LN
Telephone: 0141 300 1100
Web site: *www.show.scot.nhs.uk/scieh*

Web sites

Department of Health Travel Advice (for the general public)
Web site: *www.doh.gov.uk/traveladvice*

TRAVAX (information service for professionals – on subscription, run by SCIEH)
Web site: *www.axl.co.uk/scieh/*

World Health Organisation
Web site: *www.who.int/home-page/*

Chapter 12
Sexual Health

The patients have the added advantage of continuity of care when a practice provides a comprehensive range of services. Practice nurses see patients of all ages and have the opportunity to promote sexual health as a part of healthy living. There are several aspects to sexual health:

- Having a positive sense of sexual identity and self-worth
- Being able to sustain mutually satisfying relationships in which both partners feel secure enough to express personal needs or wishes
- Preventing unwanted pregnancies
- Avoiding sexually transmitted diseases.

Sexual identity

Sexual identity involves more than male or female gender (which is usually decided *in utero*). Practice nurses need to be aware of cultural differences and the variety of ways in which sexuality can be expressed. Ideas of masculinity and femininity undergo periodic changes. In areas of high male unemployment, men who previously had a dominant role in the household, may lose their sense of self-worth as their wives find employment instead. In other areas women expect equality as a right, but this change in the balance of power can cause anxiety for men. Some women can be frustrated in their attempts to achieve their full potential, while some men feel inadequate when faced by assertive females.

Conflict can occur in immigrant families, when young people brought up in the West rebel against the cultural expectations of their families. Forced marriages and different attitudes to divorce can cause problems within families. Female genital mutilation is still practised in some African and Middle Eastern countries. It has been illegal in the UK since 1985 but the law has not been rigorously upheld. Female genital mutilation could pose child protection issues for doctors and nurses working with refugees and asylum seekers who still adopt this custom[1].

In a predominantly heterosexual society, minority groups have had to campaign hard for equality. Attitudes to homosexuality have been changing gradually, but a great deal of homophobia still exists. Anybody who feels uncomfortable dealing with gay men or lesbians should examine the reasons, and find ways to ensure that homosexual patients are not disadvantaged. The need for sexual health education and advice for patients with learning disabilities has only been recognised relatively recently and attempts have been made in some areas to tailor services to those needs.

Sexuality has been a neglected area of nurse education and many nurses do not feel comfortable discussing issues relating to sex. Every nurse needs to have come to terms with his/her own feelings before being able to help patients. The degree of involvement in sexual health issues will vary with the knowledge and expertise of individual nurses.

Relationships

Nurses should be aware of the many ways in which patients can experience problems:

- Ignorance about the way the body functions, or how the emotions can affect sexual functioning.
- Lack of self-esteem – not being able to say 'no', or to refuse unsafe sex.
- Conflict between personal desires and the pressures to conform to the cultural norm.
- Effects of illness, drugs, or disability. Carers can experience a role conflict when expected to be both nurse and lover. Medication such as beta-blockers can cause impotence. Patients recovering from a heart attack may fear a recurrence with any exertion. Patients with severe arthritis, paraplegia or other disabilities, may have practical problems with sexual performance.
- Loneliness in patients without a partner can lead to depression and a lack of purpose in life.
- Ageism – when people over a certain age are no longer thought to need a sexual relationship.

Patients with some of these problems may need specialised help but a practice nurse who recognises the existence of the problem can offer appropriate information, counselling, or referral elsewhere as appropriate.

Education for nurses

The family planning and reproductive sexual health care course approved by the National Boards (ENB 903 in England) provides a broad education in issues concerned with sexual health, fertility and contraception. Other specialised courses can be undertaken in sexually transmitted diseases, fertility care and psychosexual counselling. The advanced family planning course (ENB A08) allows experienced family planning nurses to develop specialist knowledge and skills. The term *family planning* is still widely used to cover all aspects of reproductive health. Family planning nurses are required to keep their knowledge and skills up to date. The RCN Sexual Health Forum runs study days and issues a newsletter for members. The FPA (formerly the Family Planning Association), produces a wide range of useful literature, runs courses for health and social care professionals and provides advice and information.

Family planning

Family planning should not be considered as an exclusively female concern. Couples may attend the surgery together to discuss contraception, preparation for pregnancy, infertility, or sterilisation. Some patients prefer to visit a family planning clinic because it offers anonymity. Many clinics are now run by family planning nurses, who can prescribe within the terms of patient group directions. Adolescents often fear that the GP will tell their parents about the consultation[2]. In many areas, special under-eighteen centres have been developed for young people at suitable venues, in order to address this concern.

However, practice nurses can offer reassurance that their service is strictly confidential and will not be discussed with anyone without the consent of the patient. The law on the provision of contraceptive advice to children under 16 was clarified as a result of the judgement in the Gillick case[3]. Parental responsibility should not be undermined and whenever possible the young person should be persuaded to tell a parent or guardian but if, for example, family relationships have broken down, a doctor or nurse would not be acting unlawfully if the young person:

- Was sufficiently mature to understand all the implications
- Would not allow a parent to know that contraceptive advice was being sought
- Would be very likely to have sexual intercourse without contraception.

Since that time, young people have been assessed for what has become known as Gillick competence.

Assessment of the patient

A number of aspects need to be considered when a doctor or nurse first sees any patient for sexual health advice:

- General medical history – to identify any contraindications to specific methods of contraception
- Obstetric and gynaecological history – including menses, pregnancies, rubella status, cervical screening
- Personal history – because smoking, lifestyle or relationships may influence the choice of method

- Family history – in case the patient may have an inherited susceptibility to cardiovascular disease, diabetes or cancer
- Measurement of BP, weight and height as part of the general health assessment (also because hormone contraception can cause weight gain and elevation of the blood pressure)
- Cervical screening as appropriate
- Pelvic and breast examination if clinically indicated.

The criteria for contraception

There is no perfect method of contraception. The points to consider when choosing a method include:

- The safety of the method and any potential health risks
- The efficacy and reliability of the method
- The acceptability to both partners
- The availability – where and how easily it can be obtained
- The cost, if any.

Counselling

Patients should be able to make their own decisions after receiving adequate information and the chance to explore any fears or anxieties. It is important not to impose one's own values and judgements. *Your Guide to Contraception*, a leaflet produced by the FPA explains all the methods currently available, how they work, their reliability, advantages and disadvantages and other relevant information. The leaflet can be used as a basis for discussion when helping patients to compare the different methods.

Methods of contraception available

Oral contraception

There are many formulations of the pill but they can be grouped into two distinct types:

- The combined oral contraceptive pill
- The progestogen only pill.

The doctor or FP nurse will prescribe the appropriate type of pill after a discussion with the patient and consideration of any contraindications.

The combined oral contraceptive pill (COC)   COCs contain oestrogen and progestogen and act by inhibiting ovulation. A pill is taken daily for 21 days followed by seven pill-free days. A withdrawal bleed usually occurs during this week. If any pills are missed, especially at the beginning or end of a packet (to lengthen the number of pill-free days), then ovulation and pregnancy could occur. (See Figure 12.1 Missed pill guidelines.) The combined pill is often the first choice of younger women, for whom convenience and reliability rate highly. COCs can increase the risk of thromboembolism, so may be contra-indicated for some patients. The risk is higher in women with some inherited clotting factor defects[4]. Thrombophilia screening may be offered to women with a history of DVT in first degree relatives.

COC Pills

If less than 12 hours late taking the pill, take the pill as usual and continue normal pill-taking.

If more than 12 hours late, take the most recently missed pill, ignore any others if more than one pill missed, continue normal pill-taking and use extra precautions (condoms) for one week.

If the missed pill is one of the last seven active pills, omit the pill-free break and start the next packet. If using an ED preparation, discard the placebo pills and start the next packet. Use extra precautions for one week.

If late in restarting after the pill-free week, or two or more pills missed within the first seven days of a new packet, emergency contraception is recommended.

If more than four pills missed in the second or third week of the packet, emergency contraception is recommended.

POP Pills

Should be regarded as missed if more than three hours late in taking POP pill.

If more than three hours late, take the most recently missed pill and continue normal pill-taking. Use extra precautions for one week.

If unprotected intercourse occurs when one or more pills are missed, emergency contraception is recommended.

Figure 12.1   Missed pill guidelines.

Phasic pills contain varying hormone strengths which are intended to mimic the natural cycle. They have been thought to give a better bleeding pattern but more pill-taking errors can occur and the evidence for their use is inconclusive. Every Day (ED) pill packets contain seven placebo pills to be taken after the 21 active pills. They are useful for patients who forget to restart a packet after a week's break but the pills must be taken in the correct order. Mistakes are easier if two packets need to be taken without a pill-free break.

The progestogen only pill (POP)   POPs work mainly by thickening the cervical mucus to make it impenetrable to sperm, inhibiting transportation in the Fal-lopian tubes and by making the endometrium unsuitable for implantation.

Therefore, the pills must be taken at the same time (or within three hours) every day, without a break, in order to maintain these physiological effects. POPs may also inhibit ovulation in some women. The bleeding pattern may be more erratic than with the COC pill, and weight gain or mood changes may make the method less well-tolerated. POPs do not carry a thromboembolic risk, so are more suitable for older women, heavy smokers and others who cannot be prescribed the combined pill[5]. POPs can also be taken by breastfeeding mothers.

Emergency contraception

Emergency hormone contraception can be prescribed up to 72 hours after unprotected intercourse, but it is likely to be more effective if taken within 24 hours of the accident[6]. The patient needs to understand why she should be honest about any other unprotected sexual intercourse during that menstrual cycle; she could already be pregnant, in which case, hormone emergency contraception would not work. Nurses may supply the tablets under a patient group direction, but it is essential to adhere to the terms of the PGD and to ensure there are no contraindications to the treatment.

Levonorgestrel 750 mg has been shown to be more reliable that the combined pill (PC4) used in the past and subsequently withdrawn from sale[7]. Levonorgestrel can be prescribed by a GP, issued by a nurse under a PGD or be purchased OTC from a pharmacy. The total dose is two tablets; one to be taken as soon as possible and the second after 12 hours. Patients should be advised to time the first pill so that it does not necessitate having to wake up at an unreasonable time to take the second one. The pills are less likely to cause symptoms of nausea but, if vomiting does occur within three hours of taking it, the dose will need to be repeated. The tablets will not cause a withdrawal bleed but the patient should be warned that the next period could be earlier or later than expected. Other information and advice should cover the need:

- To use a barrier method until the next period
- To consider suitable methods of contraception for the longer term
- To return to the surgery if low abdominal pain or heavy bleeding develops, which could indicate an ectopic pregnancy
- To attend for follow up after 3–4 weeks if the period is abnormally light, heavy or does not start at all.

A written information sheet would help to reinforce any verbal advice given.

A copper-bearing intrauterine device (IUD) may be fitted as an alternative to hormone emergency contraception, if there has been more than one episode of unprotected intercourse or more than 72 hours have elapsed since the last episode. An IUD may be inserted up to five days after the likeliest date of ovulation if unprotected intercourse occurred more than five days before[8]. The method is considered to be more reliable than hormone emergency contraception and should be considered if the avoidance of pregnancy is essential. However, it is an invasive procedure which carries other risks. The contra-indications and side effects are the same as for IUDs fitted for regular contra-ception (see below, IUDs).

Oral contraceptive routines

Each practice should have agreed guidelines both for working with patients who need oral contraception for the first time, and those having follow-up appointments.

First-time pill users   New pill users require education about:

- How the pill works and affects the body
- How to take the pill and when to start (day one of cycle will give immediate contraceptive protection)
- What to do if a pill is missed
- How diarrhoea and vomiting or some medicines and antibiotics can prevent the pill from being absorbed; so extra precautions, such as condoms, are needed
- How to recognise any abnormal effects and when to contact the surgery
- The risk of sexually transmitted diseases and the use of condoms for pro-tection.

There is too much information for a patient to remember after being told once, so appropriate instruction sheets are needed as well. The doctor or nurse must check that the patient understands the information given.

Patients already taking the pill   New pill users should return after three months, when BP, weight and bleeding can be recorded, and any problems or worries discussed. Established pill users require a pill-check every six months to one year, depending on the practice policy. Regular cervical smears should be offered once a woman has been sexually active or reached 20 years of age. The patient's knowledge and understanding of her pill use should be checked to ensure that no essential information has been forgotten or misunderstood.

Barrier methods

The diaphragm   The diaphragm is a fairly commonly prescribed barrier method. Diaphragms are made of thin latex rubber, in a range of sizes from 60 mm to 90 mm in diameter. Each one has a flexible wire inside the rim to make it fit comfortably in the vagina. The cervix is covered by the diaphragm with the rim positioned in the posterior fornix and behind the pubic rim in the vagina. Flat spring and arcing spring diaphragms are the only diaphragms available on prescription.

The cervical cap These fit over the cervix and are held in place by suction. Although caps are less commonly prescribed in general practice, they can be useful for patients with lax pelvic floor muscles or women prone to cystitis when using a diaphragm.

Diaphragms and caps should to be used in conjunction with a spermicide. The patient needs to be taught by a family planning trained nurse or doctor. A plastic model of the female reproductive tract, specially designed to receive a diaphragm, is an excellent visual aid. The teaching should cover:

- How to locate the cervix
- How and when to insert the diaphragm or cap and to check that the cervix is covered
- To use extra spermicide if more than three hours have elapsed since the device was inserted, or intercourse last occurred
- How and when to remove the device (six hours must have elapsed after intercourse)
- How to look after the cap and check for any damage or perishing (any contact with oil-based products will cause the rubber to perish)
- When to return for a check or refitting (annual checks or if a significant weight change or pregnancy occurs)
- How to obtain emergency contraception if needed.

A diaphragm or cervical cap is a popular method with many women for whom the pill is unacceptable or contraindicated. The method may not be suitable for a woman who is unhappy about feeling her cervix or inserting the device. Some patients may develop an allergy to the spermicide and thus have to use an alternative method.

Male and female condoms Condoms have had significant publicity since the advent of HIV and AIDS. Free condoms are issued at family planning and GUM clinics but, unfortunately, too few general practices are able to provide them. Patients need to be reminded about the protection condoms can offer against sexually transmitted diseases as well as pregnancy, and of the correct way to apply a condom. The following points are essential:

- Make sure the condom has been stored properly and is not past its sell-by date
- Open the foil wrap carefully so the condom is not damaged
- Expel the air from the teat at the end of the condom to allow room for the ejaculate
- Roll the condom onto the erect penis before any contact with the partner's genital area takes place
- Hold the condom in place and withdraw the penis before it becomes flaccid after ejaculation
- Dispose of used condoms safely (wrap it in a tissue and place in a bin: do not flush it down the toilet)

- Make sure a female partner knows about emergency contraception if a condom fails.

The female condom is a more recent innovation which has not achieved widespread popularity. The condom is a polyurethane sac with a polythene ring inside to help the insertion of the condom into the vagina, and a fixed ring around the opening which lies over the labia. It provides some protection against genital herpes and other sexually transmitted diseases. The condoms can be bought in pharmacies but are expensive and can only be used once.

The intrauterine device (IUD)

The method, also known as the coil, involves the insertion of a small plastic and copper device into the uterus where it acts by inhibiting the passage of sperm and preventing the implantation of a fertilised ovum in the endometrium. They can stay in place for up to five years, or until the menopause in women over forty years, in the absence of any problems[9]. Fine nylon threads, attached to the end of the IUD, pass through the cervix to aid the removal of the device.

The IUD has always been considered to be more suitable for multiparous women because the slightly increased risk of pelvic infection could threaten the future fertility of women without children but recent research suggests that IUDs are safe for nulliparous women[10]. However, insertion can be more difficult when the cervix has never been dilated in labour. It is good practice to take swabs from all patients, to rule out any infection, before inserting an IUD[11]. The device must be inserted by a family planning doctor or a specially trained nurse. The ideal time for insertion is at the end of a menstrual period. The practice nurse will usually prepare the equipment, assist as needed, and look after the patient throughout the procedure (see Chapter 5). Patients can imagine tremendous horrors, so it is worth keeping some unsterile IUDs to demonstrate to patients what the coil looks like, where it is put, and how it works.

The patient needs to have clear information about the possible immediate and later effects, and when to consult the doctor. Any slight abdominal discomfort usually settles within a day or two but an urgent appointment is needed if there is persistent pain in the fortnight following insertion. If low abdominal pain, fever or vaginal discharge occur there may be some pelvic infection, which requires treatment.

Gynefix   Unlike the rigid IUDs, Gynefix is a flexible device consisting of six copper beads strung on a suture, which is attached to the fundus of the uterus. Special training is needed to insert and remove the device, which can stay in place for five years.

The intrauterine system (IUS, Mirena)   The IUS looks like a conventional IUD but instead of copper wound around the stem, it has a sleeve containing levonorgestrel, which is released in minute quantities every day. Levonorgestrel acts locally to thicken the cervical mucus and to prevent proliferation of the endometrium. This, in turn, can make bleeding so light that the IUS can be used to control menorrhagia[12]. Patients can get spotting and irregular bleeding when the IUS is first inserted but bleeding may eventually become non-existent as the progestogen inhibits ovulation.

Contraceptive hormone injections

Injectable contraceptives have become very popular with some patients. Depot medroxyprogesterone acetate (DMPA) is most commonly used. It is given as Depo-Provera 150 mg by deep intramuscular injection every 12 weeks and provides immediate contraceptive cover if started before day five of the cycle. The injection can also be given within five days of a miscarriage or abortion, or five to six weeks after childbirth. Depo-Provera suppresses ovulation and as with other progestogens, makes the cervical mucus impenetrable to sperm and prevents proliferation of the endometrium.

Norethisterone enanthate (Noristerat) is an oily injection licensed for short-term contraception. It lasts for eight weeks and may be repeated once only. There are few indications for its use in general practice; perhaps when a patient needs to avoid pregnancy following immunisation against rubella, or is waiting for a negative sperm count after a partner's vasectomy.

Nurses giving depot contraception under a patient group direction must observe the exclusions to administration and seek medical advice when necessary. Nurses who give injections prescribed by a GP should have a practice procedure to follow. The hormone cannot be removed once it has been injected, so patients must be made aware of possible side effects so they know what to expect and can give informed consent to the procedure. The following points need to be remembered:

- Weight gain can be a problem for some patients[13]. Advice can be given about eating sensibly.
- Mood swings or depression akin to premenstrual syndrome may occur.
- Heavy, prolonged or irregular bleeding in the months after the first injection will usually settle, and amenorrhoea occurs frequently, as a result of the suppression of ovulation.
- Delay in return to fertility can occur. It can take up to a year for periods to recommence once injections are stopped.
- Bone density may be affected if adolescent women are given DMPA injections[14]. Maximum bone density is normally achieved during the teenage years. More research is needed into the long-term effects but to date, the evidence suggests that for most patients, the residual effects of DMPA on post-menopausal bone density are small and unlikely to increase the risk of fractures in the post-menopausal years[15].

Patients should be made aware that the effect of the Depo-Provera injection may start to wear off after 12 weeks but that it can be given earlier if the patient will be away on the due date, for any reason. Advice should be sought if a patient presents more than 12 weeks and five days after her last injection.

Progestogen implants

Norplant   This product consists of six rods containing a slow release progestogen to be implanted under the skin of the upper arm and was withdrawn in 1999 but a few patients could have them *in situ* until 2004. Problems with removal of the rods and the adverse publicity contributed to the withdrawal of Norplant by the manufacturer.

Implanon   This is the only implant available in the UK now. It consists of a single rod inserted subcutaneously, which releases etonogestrel over a three year period. At the end of three years the rod should be removed and replaced. The method has been found to be a reliable method of contraception but weight gain and irregular bleeding have been common side effects[16].

Natural methods

Religious or personal reasons may lead some couples to opt for natural family planning. A high level of motivation is required and special teaching is essential. Couples can avoid intercourse once they have learned to identify the fertile time each month. Various methods may be used, often in combination:

- Calendar – keeping records of the menstrual cycle. Ovulation occurs 14 days before the menstrual period starts but cannot be predicted accurately in advance, even with a regular cycle.
- Temperature – very careful recordings of the body temperature each day, using a special fertility thermometer, to identify the slight temperature rise which occurs at ovulation (febrile illness will nullify the readings).
- Cervical mucus can be used to recognise the fertile time because the consistency and amount of the mucus changes around the time of ovulation to facilitate the entry of sperm.
- Commercially available test kits detect ovulation by the surge in luteinising hormone, but do not yet predict ovulation early enough to be reliable for contraception.
- The Persona device, originally marketed in 1996 as being as reliable as condoms, was subject to a Medical Devices Agency adverse incident report and found to have a higher failure rate than the manufacturers claimed. However, it is said to be useful as a test-based method of natural family planning[17].

The success or failure of natural methods relies on being able to predict ovulation accurately so that intercourse is avoided for at least five days before and three days afterwards.

Male and female sterilisation

Sterilisation is the ultimate contraception. It should be regarded as permanent even though advances in microsurgery might make reversal possible. Couples who have completed their families may opt for this method, but with divorce and second marriages now so common, they need to consider all the possible eventualities before reaching a decision about sterilisation.

Vasectomy   Sterilisation for the male entails cutting the spermatic cord just as it enters the inguinal canal after leaving the scrotum. It is an easy operation which can be performed under local anaesthetic as an outpatient. Some GPs will perform vasectomies in the surgery. The patient should be advised not to undertake strenuous physical activity for a few days, in order to minimise any possibility of bruising around the operation site. The following points should be emphasised when discussing this method of sterilisation with patients:

- It is permanent, but not until two consecutive sperm counts are negative
- There will be no adverse effect on erection, sexual performance, or ejaculation
- As the majority of the ejaculate is made up of secretions from the prostate and other glands the patient will notice little change after the operation.

Semen samples are required monthly for 3–4 months after the operation. Contraceptive precautions must be continued until two consecutive samples contain no sperm. At one time there was some concern about an increased risk of prostatic cancer after vasectomy but no evidence has been found to support this[18].

Female sterilisation   A woman is sterilised by cutting or clipping the Fallopian tubes so that the ovum cannot pass down them into the uterus. The vast majority of female sterilisations are carried out under general anaesthetic using a laparoscope in a day surgery unit. Patients may experience some discomfort after the procedure but this rarely last more than a few days. The practice nurse may be required to remove the sutures from the small abdominal incision sites.

Education

Any method of contraception can fail if the user does not learn everything he or she needs to know about using the method safely. Doctors and nurses who provide family planning services need to have enough time, appropriate visual aids, and be able to choose suitable teaching styles for each patient.

Administrative aspects

Patients who receive contraceptive advice or treatment by a GP or family planning nurse must also have regular reviews. This means that the patient's record must show what method is being used and when the next check is due. The GP can claim item of service fees for providing family planning services, so the claims must be completed, usually by computer, to ensure that practice income is not lost. The following is a list of possible claims:

- FP1001 is claimed annually for all patients who have been offered contraception or advice about contraceptive methods.
- FP1002 is a fee claim for the insertion of an IUD or IUS. Thereafter an annual fee is claimed on FP1001 for the annual IUD check. An FP1002 claim can only be made once in a year, even if an IUD is fitted more than once in that year.
- FP1003 is a fee claim for giving contraceptive advice to a temporary patient. Patients are allowed to consult any GP for contraceptive advice without having to be registered at that practice. This can be useful when a patient is embarrassed about seeing a GP who is an old family friend. It is important for reception staff to be aware of this ruling, so that they do not turn patients away.

Termination of pregnancy

It is vital that nobody enters a sexual relationship with the attitude that 'if anything goes wrong an abortion can be arranged'. Apart from the undesirability of using termination as a form of contraception, there are health risks which include:

- A higher incidence of pelvic inflammatory disease
- Cervical incompetence in future wanted pregnancies
- The usual operative risks of anaesthesia and of haemorrhage
- The psychological consequences.

The decision of a doctor to refer a woman for a termination will depend on a number of factors which can only be taken into account after careful discussion and counselling. The law requires that a statement be completed by two doctors (preferably the GP and the gynaecologist) who have to state that the patient falls into one of four categories:

- The continuation of the pregnancy would involve risk to the life of the pregnant woman greater than if the pregnancy was terminated
- The continuance of the pregnancy would involve risk of injury to the physical or mental health of the pregnant woman greater than if the pregnancy was terminated

- The continuance of the pregnancy would involve risk of injury to the physical or mental health of the pregnant woman or any existing child(ren) of her family greater than if the pregnancy was terminated
- There is substantial risk that if the child was born it would suffer from such physical and mental abnormalities as to be severely handicapped[19].

The termination itself may be performed within the NHS or privately. (Abortion is not available in Northern Ireland, except in very exceptional circumstances.) All patients who have a termination must be encouraged to undertake ways of preventing further unwanted pregnancies. The moral and ethical aspects of termination have not been considered here because each reader will have his or her own opinion on this emotive subject. However, the UKCC requires nurses to promote and safeguard the interest and well-being of their patients and clients, and to ensure that no act or omission within the nurse's sphere of responsibility is detrimental to a patient's interest, condition or safety[20].

Sexually transmitted diseases

The risks of acquiring a sexually transmitted disease (STD) should be explained when discussing contraception or sexual health issues. *Chlamydia*, genital warts, herpes, HIV and hepatitis B can all be transmitted sexually; not just syphilis and gonorrhoea. A patient with symptoms of a sexually transmitted disease should be advised to attend the genito-urinary medicine (GUM) clinic, where the facilities exist for prompt diagnosis and treatment, as well as counselling and contact-tracing. It is not uncommon for patients to have more than one sexually transmitted infection at the same time, which makes a full sexual health screen so important. Practice nurses can help patients by providing information about the clinic times and location and reassuring patients about the confidentiality maintained there.

Chlamydia

Chlamydia is a disease caused by the bacterium *Chlamydia trachomatis*, which is primarily transmitted through sexual intercourse. The urethra and rectum may be infected and transmission of genital discharge to the eyes can cause conjunctivitis. The infant of a mother with *Chlamydia* may be born prematurely, have a chlamydial eye infection or develop pneumonia after delivery.

Symptoms

Both men and women can be asymptomatic and thus be unaware of the problem.

Men may experience burning during micturition, or discharge from the penis. In the longer term, they may develop epididymitis or Reiter's syndrome (an autoimmune condition affecting the joints and the eyes), or fertility problems.

Women may experience burning on micturition or an abnormal vaginal discharge. Pelvic inflammatory disease, leading to infertility, is a serious consequence of *Chlamydia* infection. For this reason, a great deal is talked about routinely screening young sexually-active women for *Chlamydia*. As yet there is no national screening programme and local policies should be followed. There is some evidence that urine testing for *Chlamydia* in general practice can detect a significant number of people with *Chlamydia* but public awareness needs to be raised about the risks from undiagnosed infection[21].

Genital warts

Genital warts, caused by the human papilloma virus (HPV), are usually transmitted sexually and may have a long incubation period from infection to the development of warts. They may be difficult to see, or be flat or cauliflower-shaped in appearance. They are not usually painful but can cause intense irritation. They may be found on the shaft of the penis, on or under the foreskin in males; around the vulva or in the vagina in females. Patients of either sex may have warts around the anus, and the mouth may be infected through oral sex. Treatment may be by the application of podophyllin, cryocautery, laser or surgical excision. HPV is recognised as a cause of cervical neoplasia[22]. Women with genital warts must be advised to have regular smear tests.

Genital herpes

Genital herpes is caused by the herpes simplex virus (HSV). There are two types, HSV-1 usually causes cold sores on the mouth (see Chapter 8), although cold sores can also be transmitted to the genital areas through oral sex. HSV-2, which causes the typical blisters of genital herpes, is primarily transmitted sexually and usually affects the genital areas. HSV-2 can be transmitted to the mouth and throat through oral sex. Patients need to be aware of how the virus is spread so they can:

- Adopt good hygiene practices to avoid spread to other parts of the body
- Practice safer sex and also avoid the risk of infection through oral sex
- Avoid sex when the herpes is present or developing.

Topical or systemic antivirals may be helpful in the very early stage of herpes. The most severe symptoms usually occur with the first outbreak but recurrent attacks can occur when the dormant virus is reactivated in response to stress or other factors. Immunocompromised patients may develop very severe herpes.

Hepatitis B (see Chapter 4)

Patients at risk of contracting hepatitis B through sexual activity should be offered immunisation in addition to information about the disease and the need to practice safe(r) sex.

Human immunodeficiency virus infection (HIV)

HIV infection, like hepatitis B, can be transmitted through blood or body fluids. This may be via an infected needle, contact with mucous membranes or through unprotected sexual intercourse. The majority of people with HIV infection are asymptomatic. The progression of the disease to Acquired Immune Deficiency Syndrome (AIDS) varies from person to person. Persistent generalised lymphadenopathy, or generalised symptoms related to immune deficiency, such as severe diarrhoea and weight loss, fatigue, night sweats, candidiasis, and herpes may first point to a diagnosis of HIV infection. Opportunistic diseases which would normally be overcome by the T4 cells can become life-threatening. *Pneumocystis carinii* pneumonia (PCP), cytomegalo-virus infection, tuberculosis, and Karposi's sarcoma are diagnostic of AIDS in HIV positive patients. Neurological involvement can lead to loss of motor or sensory function and dementia.

Better drugs and technology are allowing many patients to live for years with HIV infection but they still require support and kindness. Voluntary organisations exist for HIV positive men, women, children and partners, as well as members of ethnic groups and religions. Practice nurses can assist by treating patients with HIV as any other patients who need help or advice, and by educating other people about the disease. The local HIV/AIDS adviser will provide any extra training needed.

The spread of HIV infection is linked to the incidence of other sexually transmitted diseases like syphilis and gonorrhoea. When the number of cases increases it shows that the message about safe(r) sex is not getting through or is being ignored. Practice nurses may have the opportunity to spread the message when discussing contraception with patients, or when giving travel advice. Safe sex relates to activities such as kissing, fondling, massaging, masturbation, or the use of sex toys, which do not involve penetrative intercourse. Safer sex is the term used to describe vaginal, oral or anal sex protected by an appropriate condom[23]. There is a wide variety of condoms available. Extra strong ones are necessary for anal intercourse.

> ## Suggestions for reflection on practice
>
> How good is your sexual health service?
>
> - Is your knowledge up to date?
> - Do all patient groups access the service?
> - Can patients get emergency contraception promptly?
> - How do you know what patients have understood from a consultation?
> - How do you know if the patients are satisfied with the service?

Further reading

Royal College of Nursing (2000) *Sexuality and Sexual Health in Nursing Practice*. Royal College of Nursing, London.

References

1. British Medical Association Guidance (revised 2001) *Female Genital Mutilation: Caring for patients and child protection*. *www.bma.org.uk/public/ethics.nsf* (accessed 6/10/01).
2. Burrack, R. (2000) Young teenagers' attitudes towards general practice and their provision of sexual health care. *British Journal of General Practice*, **50** (456), 550–54.
3. House of Lords ruling (1985) *Gillick v. West Norfolk and Wisbech Area Health Authority*. HMSO, London.
4. Hannaford, P. (2000) Cardiovascular events associated with different combined oral contraceptives. A review of current data. *Drug Safety*, **22**, 361–71.
5. British Medical Association, Royal Pharmaceutical Society of Great Britain (2001) *British National Formulary*, **41**, 7.3.2.1.
6. Piaggio, G., von Hertzen, H., Grimes, D. & Van Look, P. (1999) Timing of emergency contraception with levonorgestrel or the Yupze regimen. Task Force on Post-ovulatory Methods of Fertility Regulation. *Lancet*, **352** (9126), 721.
7. Cheng, L., Gulmezoglu, A., Ezcurra, E. & Van Look, P. (2000) Interventions for emergency contraception (Cochrane Review) In: *The Cochrane Library*, **21**, 1–15. Update Software, Oxford.
8. Faculty of Family Planning and Reproductive Healthcare (2000) Emergency contraception: recommendations for clinical practice. *British Journal of Family Planning*, **26**, 93–6.
9. Tacchi, D. (1990) Long-term use of copper intrauterine devices. *Lancet*, **336**, 182.
10. Hubacher, D., Lara-Ricalde, R., Taylor, D., Guerra-Infante, F. & Guzman-Rodriguez, R. (2001) Use of copper intrauterine devices and the risk of tubal infertility among nulligravid women. *New England Journal of Medicine*, **345** (8), 561–7.
11. Templeton, A. (ed.) (1996) *The Prevention of Pelvic Infection*. Royal College of Obstetricians and Gynaecologists, London.

12. Stewart, A., Cummins, C., Gold, L., Jordan, R. & Phillips, W. (2001) The effectiveness of the levonorgestrel-releasing intrauterine system in menorrhagia: a systematic review. *British Journal of Obstetrics and Gynaecology*, **108** (1), 74–86.

13. Bigrigg, A., Evans, A., Gbolade, B. *et al.* (1999) Depo-provera. Position paper on clinical use, effectiveness and side effects. *British Journal of Family Planning*, **25** (2), 69–76.

14. Kass-Wolff, J. (2001) Bone loss in adolescents using Depo-Provera. *Journal of the Society of Pediatric Nursing*, **6** (1), 21–31.

15. Orr-Walker, B., Evans, M., Ames, R., Clearwater, J., Cundy, T. & Reid, I. (1998) The effect of past use of the injectable contraceptive depot medroxyprogesterone acetate on bone mineral density in normal post-menopausal women. *Clinical Endocrinology*, **49** (5), 615–18.

16. Edwards, J.E. & Moore, A. (1999) Implanon: a review of clinical studies. *British Journal of Family Planning*, **4**, 3–16.

17. Tucker, D.E. (1998) Persona Contraceptive – MDA report. *www.womens-health.co.uk/persona* (accessed 16/8/01).

18. Stanford, J., Wicklund, K., McNight, B., Daling, J. & Brewer, M. (1999) Vasectomy and risk of prostate cancer. *Cancer Epidemiology Biomarkers and Prevention*, **8** (10), 881–6.

19. Great Britain, Parliament (1967) *The Abortion Act 1967*. HMSO, London.

20. United Kingdom Central Council for Nurses, Midwives and Health Visitors (1992) *Code of Professional Conduct*, para. 2. UKCC, London.

21. Tobin, C., Aggarwal, R., Clarke, J., Chown, R. & King, D. (2001) *Chlamydia trachomatis*: opportunistic screening in primary care. *British Journal of General Practice*, **51**, 565–6.

22. Wolf, J. and Ramirez, P. (2001) The molecular biology of cervical cancer. *Cancer Investigation*, **19** (6), 621–9.

23. Everett, S. (1997) Contraception. In: *Women's Sexual Health* (ed. G. Andrews), pp. 73–4. Bailliere Tindall, London.

Useful addresses and web sites

FPA (formerly the Family Planning Association)
Web site: *www.fpa.org.uk*

National AIDS Helpline (24 hours)
Telephone: 0800 567123

Chapter 13
Women's Health

The expectation by society that women should care for others such as partners, children and elderly parents, can mean, in some situations, that they have little time left to care for themselves. A practice nurse who shows a friendly concern can allow women to put their own interests first, for a while. Regular well-woman checks have been offered since the national cervical screening programme was established. However, this relies on the postal system so travellers, homeless women or those not registered with the NHS may not receive an invitation to attend. Well-woman screening involves factors related to the female reproductive function in addition to the general health screening outlined in Chapter 9, and should involve much more than cervical cytology. A thorough history is needed to ensure that every patient receives the appropriate care and advice.

Menstruation

Nurses should be aware of the range of normal menstrual cycles for different women in order to recognise any abnormalities of menstruation. There may be considerable variations in cycle length and menstrual flow but an average normal pattern can be considered as:

- The start of menstrual periods (menarche) age 10–13 years. They may be irregular at first but settle into a regular cycle by about 16 years.
- A menstrual cycle of approximately 28 days with bleeding over 4–5 days. (The first day of bleeding is calculated as day 1 of the cycle.)
- The cessation of menstrual periods (menopause) between about 48–54 years. However, some women could have a normal menopause at an earlier or a later age. Premature menopause is the term used when it occurs before the age of 40.

A practice nurse can help a woman with concerns about menstruation by:

- Getting the patient to give a clear outline of the problem
- Checking on the patient's knowledge and understanding of menstruation

- Showing her how to keep a menstrual chart and encouraging her to consult the GP with it, if necessary
- Giving practical advice for dealing with discomfort, and using appropriate sanitary protection
- Referring the patient to the GP for any problem needing medical investigation or treatment.

Young women should be taught why menstruation is a normal event rather than a curse, but women who do have problems with menstruation deserve sympathetic understanding.

Dysmenorrhoea

Painful periods cause misery for some women each month. Exercise can often relieve the cramp-like pain of normal periods, and mild analgesics may help. Mefanamic acid, flufenamic acid or the contraceptive pill may be prescribed for more severe pain. Secondary dysmenorrhoea, requiring medical investigation, can be caused by an IUD, pelvic inflammatory disease, endometriosis or fibroids.

Menorrhagia

Heavy, regular menstrual bleeding over several consecutive cycles, can be distressing and embarrassing to the patient and lead to iron-deficiency anaemia. The extent of the problem needs to be assessed and abnormal pathology ruled out. Patients can be asked to record the number of pads or tampons used, the frequency of change and any clots passed. Heavy, irregular bleeding may develop in the peri-menopausal years but post-coital or inter-menstrual bleeding could be indicative of more serious problems. A haemoglobin estimation is recommended to check for anaemia and a patient with menorrhagia should be examined by a GP. A levonorgestrel-releasing intra-uterine system might be inserted to control menorrhagia, as an alternative to hysterectomy[1].

Amenorrhoea

Primary amenorrhoea – delay in the onset of periods may be the result of a congenital physiological factor, such as the absence of a uterus or vagina, an endocrine disturbance, or an eating disorder.

Secondary amenorrhoea – the absence of menstruation for six months in a woman who has previously had periods, is most commonly caused by pregnancy; a cause which should always be considered, and tested for if pregnancy is feasible. Breastfeeding may delay the return of menstruation after pregnancy.

Other factors include: anxiety, moving to a new environment, examination stress, strenuous exercise, eating disorders, or endocrine problems. Secondary amenorrhoea can result from hormone contraceptive use and patients should be made aware of this when it is prescribed.

Premenstrual syndrome (PMS)

Most women experience some physiological changes during the latter half of the menstrual cycle (luteal phase). Breast tenderness or mood changes are a response to the changing hormone levels. More extreme physical or psychological symptoms are termed premenstrual syndrome. The cause is not fully understood and therapy is therefore focused more on the management of symptoms than on the underlying cause[2]. Practice nurses can help patients to talk about their problems and encourage them to keep a diary of their symptoms in relation to the menstrual cycle.

   The symptoms may be eased by a healthy diet and aerobic exercise. Coffee should be restricted because the caffeine may increase irritability. A low salt intake may reduce fluid retention and diuretics can be prescribed by the GP if necessary, although there is little evidence that water retention is related to the symptoms of PMS[3]. Pyridoxine (vitamin B6), oil of evening primrose or the contraceptive pill may help some patients although the evidence for their clinical effectiveness is limited[4].

Cervical cytology
(See Chapter 6 under diagnostic tests and investigations)

Cervical smears are taken to detect any pre-malignant changes in the cells of the cervix; cervical intra-epithelial neoplasia (CIN), which might develop into invasive cancer if not treated. The cytology report will indicate the severity of any changes and suggest when the test should be repeated, or if the patient should be referred for colposcopy. The reduction of death from cancer is one of the targets in *Saving Lives: Our Healthier Nation*[5].

Targets

GPs are paid for meeting a target of 70%, or a lower target of 50%, for cervical screening for women aged from 20 to 64 years. As with many screening activities, those most at risk can be the least likely to attend. Opportunistic screening is needed in addition to an effective call and recall system. A good administration system will help to maintain the practice income, but the prime concern should be for the welfare of women. Younger women are not included in the smear targets but regular smears may be advisable once a girl has been sexually active. However, there may be local variations in the policy on screening patients who are under 20, and women in the target group who have never been sexually active. The risks may be lower for the latter group of patients but they do still face some risk. In addition, lesbian women may contract the human papilloma virus from sex toys and thus develop cervical neoplasia[6].

Practice nurses can help to reduce the anxiety associated with cervical screening, but any nurse involved must have had the necessary theoretical and practical experience and be accountable for her practice. The degree of nurse involvement will depend on the level of knowledge and expertise. Nurses who take cervical smears must have been taught correctly and have been assessed as competent by a qualified cytology trainer. Routine bimanual pelvic examination as a screening test for ovarian cancer in asymptomatic women is not recommended[7]. Bimanual pelvic examination should only be carried out, for symptomatic women, by nurses with advanced qualifications, such as nurse practitioners or advanced family planning nurse specialists.

There are three levels of involvement:

- *Level 1*
  - Administration – checking when smears are due and reminding patients when they are seen for other purposes
  - Educating patients about cervical screening and providing appropriate literature for them to read.

- *Level 2*   As for level 1 and in addition:
  - Taking an appropriate history and completing the smear form with all the relevant personal details, and comprehensive information about previous smears
  - Taking a satisfactory cervical smear
  - Making sure the patient knows how to get the result of the test and that a contact address is known
  - Interpreting an abnormal smear result to a patient.

- *Level 3*   As for levels 1 and 2 and in addition:
  - Performing a bimanual pelvic examination to detect any tenderness or masses in the pelvic organs, if appropriate.

Laboratories vary in the terminology used to describe cervical cell changes. Nurses should ask for clarification from their local department of cytology. Smears may be described as:

- Inadequate, due to insufficient cells on the slide, cells obscured by blood or mucus, or poor fixation
- Negative – no abnormality detected
- Transformation cells not seen – the sample may not have contained cells from the squamo-columnar junction (the transformation zone), where pre-malignant changes most commonly occur
- Inflammatory – cell changes due to infection or irritation of the cervix

- Borderline dyskaryosis – some atypical cells seen
- Mild dyskariosis or CIN 1 – changes in the nuclei of some cells
- Moderate dyskariosis or CIN 2 – more marked changes in the nuclei
- Severe dyskaryosis or CIN 3 – a larger number of cells with grossly abnormal nuclei
- Malignant cells present – suggestive of invasive cancer.

Patients with borderline or mild changes will be recalled for repeat smears after six months. After three inadequate smears, three borderline results or if CIN 2 or 3 is found the patient will be referred to a gynaecology clinic for colposcopy. A leaflet produced by the Health Promotion Authority, explains to patients the procedure of colposcopy and the treatment of abnormal cells. Colposcopy means looking directly at the cervix with a special microscope attached to a vaginal speculum. The cervix is stained with iodine or acetic acid to delineate any areas of abnormality and a biopsy can be taken. Abnormal cells can be destroyed by laser cautery or cryosurgery. Occasionally a cone biopsy may be performed under general anaesthetic to remove abnormal cells which extend into the cervical canal. Patients who have had treatment for CIN must have regular smear tests and follow-up.

Breast awareness

Breast cancer is the largest single cause of death of women in the UK. The Government's Cancer Plan includes the target to reduce deaths from breast cancer[8]. Patients with several close female relatives who have had the disease may be referred to a breast unit for regular screening. All women need to understand the importance of recognising any change in their breasts and of seeking medical help quickly.

Practice nurses should not examine patients' breasts but they can teach breast awareness to their patients[9]. The principles include:

- Looking at the breasts to detect anything unusual (change in the outline, dimpling of the skin, retraction or change in a nipple). A patient should do this in front of a mirror with her arms at her side, then raised above the head, and finally with her hands pressed onto the hips, to accentuate the breast contours.

- Feeling the breast tissue. The patient should lie flat with her head on a pillow and a towel or small pillow under the shoulder to centralise the nipple of the side to be examined. Using the flat of the fingers together and working systematically around all the breast tissue and into the axilla, the breast tissue should be compressed firmly but gently against the chest wall. The nipple should be squeezed gently to see if any blood or discharge is expressed.

A doctor should be consulted immediately if any abnormality is suspected. The NHS Cancer Plan contains ambitious ideas for improving cancer services in England. There are targets for waiting times, which include a maximum of one month's wait from diagnosis to treatment. It should be emphasised however, that many breast lumps are benign.

The National Health Service Breast Screening Service

Women aged 50–64 are offered mammography every three years. The screening programme has only been in operation since 1990 but a significant number of early cancers have been detected. Nurses can encourage their patients to attend, and reassure them that the procedure only takes a few moments. It entails stripping to the waist and standing next to an X-ray machine while the breast is compressed between two special plates. This can be rather uncomfortable but only lasts for a few seconds while the X-ray is taken. If further tests are needed the patient will be invited to see the specialist at her local breast unit. Explanatory leaflets are available from regional breast screening centres.

Women aged 65–70 will be offered screening from the year 2004. Women under 50 years are not currently eligible for the programme. Women of any age who have symptoms should consult their GP because the national screening programme is only intended for asymptomatic women. Although breast screening may ultimately save lives, the unexpected diagnosis of cancer can be devastating. Such patients require skilled counselling and support.

Pre-conceptual care

Patients may ask for advice about the best ways to prepare for pregnancy. Such advice for both partners should cover lifestyle factors and the avoidance of known hazards. Healthy living means not smoking tobacco, sensible alcohol intake, having regular exercise and adequate sleep, and eating a well-balanced diet (see Chapter 9). Folic acid is important because a deficiency is thought to contribute to neural tube defects. Foods rich in folic acid include dark leafy vegetables, oranges, beans, fortified bread and breakfast cereals, beef and yeast extracts. However, increased dietary folate alone may not prevent neural tube defects[10]. Women are advised to take 0.4 mg folic acid daily while trying to conceive and during the first trimester of pregnancy.

Blood should be taken to test for rubella antibodies if a woman's immunity has not been confirmed. If a patient needs to be immunised against rubella she must be warned to avoid becoming pregnant for a minimum of one month after immunisation. Any occupational hazards to pregnant women should be identified, and a transfer may have to be considered at work. Radiation and anaesthetic gases, for example, are known to be hazardous. Any medicines a patient takes should be checked to ensure they will not harm the fetus. Some changes to medication may be necessary, so the patient should see her GP or hospital specialist. Patients who are planning to travel abroad should be made aware of any health risks, especially malaria (see Chapter 11).

It may be necessary to check the patient's understanding of the menstrual cycle and when ovulation is most likely to occur. The natural methods of contraception (see Chapter 12) can also help patients who want to conceive to recognise their fertile time. Patients with any family or personal history of a hereditary condition may be referred for genetic counselling.

Infertility

Patients who are unable to have children may consult their GP for help. Most couples will be referred to a fertility specialist, but the practice nurse may be involved with some of the fertility tests or with giving pre-conceptual health advice. Patients who embark on the stressful process of investigation and treatment of infertility will require patience and commitment. A sense of humour also helps. Specialist infertility centres must employ counsellors[11]. Practice nurses can also help by listening to patients' concerns, being sympathetic to their needs and making sure they have received all the information they require.

In vitro fertilisation (IVF) and embryo transfer

Drugs are used to stimulate several ova to ripen at once. This is carefully monitored by blood tests and ultrasound and at the appropriate time the mature eggs are collected via a laparoscope and placed in a culture medium. Specially prepared sperm collected from the partner's semen are added to the ova in the containers. Once fertilisation has occurred, the selected embryos are introduced through the cervix into the patient's uterus. Only two embryos may be introduced, in order to reduce the problems of multiple births[12]. Progesterone injections or pessaries may be given to assist the implantation. Extra embryos may be deep frozen for future use in case the pregnancy does not become established. Gamete intrafallopian transfer (GIFT) is a procedure similar to IVF except that the ova and sperm are mixed and transferred to the Fallopian tube before fertilisation.

Pregnancy

A practice nurse may be the first person to confirm a pregnancy after performing the pregnancy test. First time parents will welcome some information about what to expect. The pregnancy is counted from the first day of the last menstrual period, so the expected date of delivery can be calculated as 40 weeks from then. Special calculator discs are available for this purpose. Smoking and a high alcohol intake in pregnancy are known to be harmful. The opportunity should be taken to advise on their avoidance. Help may be offered to quit smoking. Food poisoning during pregnancy can be harmful to the fetus. Therefore, soft cheeses, pâté and undercooked meat should be avoided because of the risk of listeria infection. Raw or undercooked eggs and raw shellfish can also be a source of infection. A high intake of vitamin A can be dangerous, so pregnant women should be advised not to eat liver or large quantities of carrots[13].

Maternity care

The arrangements for maternity care can differ from area to area, so it is useful for a practice nurse to familiarise herself with the arrangements locally. Shared care between the GP, the community midwife and the obstetrician is often popular. Some GPs may provide medical cover for home confinements.

Antenatal care

A patient will attend the first antenatal clinic when she is approximately 12 weeks pregnant. The midwife obtains a full medical and obstetric history, which is summarised in the obstetric record. The patient will usually be given her own record to take to clinic appointments and the hospital during the rest of the pregnancy. The height, weight and blood pressure are recorded, and the urine is tested for glucose and albumin. A urine sample is sent for microscopy and culture if a urinary infection is suspected. Blood tests are taken for full blood count, blood group, rubella antibodies, hepatitis B, HIV and syphilis. The GP or midwife may perform a physical examination. The appropriate booking is made for home, GP unit or hospital confinement, and the patient is given a certificate of eligibility for free dental care and prescriptions.

A patient with an uncomplicated pregnancy will return for further antenatal checks at about 24 weeks and 32 weeks gestation, fortnightly until 36 weeks, and weekly thereafter. There may be local variations in the clinic intervals and investigations performed, but the following is a guide:

- 12.5 weeks: Nuchal translucency screening for chromosomal abnormalities of the fetus
- 21 weeks: Routine ultrasound scan to confirm normal growth and development of the fetus
- 28 weeks: FBC, glucose, blood group and antibodies
- 34 weeks: FBC, blood group and antibodies, if rhesus negative mother.

After 24 weeks pregnancy a certificate (MatB1) is issued, which entitles a woman to maternity benefits.

Post-natal care

The patient attends for a full post-natal examination about six weeks after confinement. The haemoglobin may be checked and rubella immunisation given, if needed. A cervical smear, if due, should be postponed until at least 12 weeks post-partum. The doctor completes the maternity claim (FP24) for providing maternity care. Contraception should be discussed at the post-natal check and appropriate arrangements made. Oral contraception can be started right away, but the progestogen-only pill must be used while the patient is breastfeeding. An IUD or diaphragm can be fitted, if preferred.

Lax pelvic floor muscles contribute to urinary incontinence and uterine prolapse. The patient should be encouraged to continue post-natal exercises to regain muscle tone and to practice pelvic floor exercises every day. Patients need to learn how to contract the pelvic floor muscles by squeezing and drawing in the muscles around the anus and vagina without tightening the buttock or abdominal muscles. The exercises should be performed up to 100 times a day; even when performing household chores. It is a good idea for all women to learn to practice pelvic floor exercises to prevent stress incontinence – not only women after childbirth[14].

Practice nurses usually have a peripheral role in ante- and post-natal care, but such contacts offer the chance to establish a good relationship so the parent will be less anxious about bringing the baby for immunisation.

Miscarriage

There can be many mishaps between conception and the delivery of a healthy infant. An anxious patient may telephone the surgery for advice. Bleeding in the early months of pregnancy may settle down, but patients need support while they wait to see what happens. Although rest probably won't affect the outcome, it can help a woman to feel she did everything possible, if the pregnancy is lost. The doctor will usually arrange an urgent ultrasound scan, but admission to hospital will be needed if the bleeding is severe. A woman with a rhesus negative blood group must be given an injection of anti-D immunoglobulin within 72 hours of a miscarriage to prevent the development of antibodies which could affect a subsequent fetus[15]. The Stillbirth and Neonatal Death Society (SANDS) provides support for bereaved parents, and information for professionals. The parents need the chance to grieve when a miscarriage or a stillbirth occurs. The importance of acknowledging the loss is now recognised, and parents are encouraged to collect mementos of the infant and to arrange a funeral ceremony[16].

Hysterectomy

The reaction of a woman after hysterectomy may range from relief at the end of miserable symptoms or the fear of pregnancy, to severe depression and grief at the supposed loss of her femininity. Physical problems, such as pain, wound infection and urinary incontinence are not uncommon and can cause distress. A patient who has had a hysterectomy because of a malignancy will continue to need regular vaginal vault smears. There are conflicting opinions about the value of preserving the ovaries when performing a hysterectomy[17]. However, pre-menopausal women whose ovaries are removed require immediate hormone replacement therapy to prevent the effects of a sudden menopause. Oestrogen replacement therapy should be offered to all women who have had a hysterectomy.

The menopause

The menopause marks the end of fertility for women as the ovaries cease to function. The decrease in oestrogen production causes physical and emotional changes, although the type and severity of symptoms can vary from one woman to another. Common symptoms include hot flushes and night sweats. The temperature regulating centre in the hypothalamus is believed to be stimulated by the increased production of gonadotrophic hormones in response to the reduced oestrogen in the circulation. Vaginal dryness and atrophy are also caused by the reduction of oestrogen. Urgency and urinary leakage can be similarly caused.

Palpitations, depression, irritability and lack of concentration are other common complaints, but caution should prevail before attributing every problem to the menopause. An unsatisfactory relationship with a partner, children leaving home, business worries, or unfulfilled ambitions can also lead to depression or sexual difficulties in middle age. A thorough history and medical examination is needed for each patient.

The longer term effects of the menopause include an increased risk of coronary heart disease and osteoporosis. Practice nurses are able to help women at the menopause by:

- Listening to their concerns
- Providing factual information about the menopause and the treatments available for symptoms
- Assessing their general health and risk factors for heart disease and osteoporosis
- Referring them to the GP for medical assessment and treatment
- Monitoring the effects of treatment.

The management of menopausal symptoms

Practice nurses should be aware of the treatments available and encourage patients to consult their doctor when necessary. The available local treatments to relieve vaginal dryness and dyspareunia include:

- Vaginal lubricants (KY jelly)
- Vaginal rehydrating gel (Feminesse, Replens)

- Local hormone replacement
- Oestriol pessaries or cream (Ortho-Gynest)
- Oestradiol vaginal tablets (Vagifem)
- Oestradiol vaginal ring (Estring).

Local oestrogen is not suitable to be used alone for more than three months by women who still have a uterus. Proliferation of the endometrium may need to be opposed by the addition of a progestogen.

Systemic treatment for the relief of symptoms or the long-term prevention of osteoporosis includes:

- Hormone replacement therapy – tablets, patches, gels or implants
- Synthetic steroids, e.g. tibolone.

Hormone replacement therapy (HRT)

Practice nurses who advise patients about the menopause need to be familiar with the arguments for and against HRT. The proponents claim that because in evolutionary terms women were not designed to live much beyond the childbearing years, HRT is needed to protect them from the problems associated with longevity. The opposing view is that a normal life event has been unnecessarily medicalised. An open mind is needed, and a willingness to keep up to date with research into the subject. HRT can relieve many of the distressing symptoms of the menopause, but there can be side effects. Therefore, patients need careful selection and regular monitoring (see *BNF*). Absolute contraindications to HRT are:

- Undiagnosed vaginal bleeding
- Pregnancy or lactation
- Cancer of the breast, of genital tract or other oestrogen-dependent tumours
- Current or previous deep vein thrombosis or other thromboembolic disorder
- Severe cardiac, renal or liver disease
- Dubin-Johnson or Rotor syndromes (congenital diseases affecting the transport of bilirubin from the liver).

Relative contraindications include:

- Previous CVS disease or hypertension
- Mild chronic liver disease or renal impairment
- Diabetes
- Obesity, prolonged immobility, trauma or surgery
- Fibroids or endometriosis.

The use of HRT for more than five years may slightly increase the risk of developing breast cancer[18]. Patients should be made aware of this. All patients over 50 on HRT should be encouraged to attend for mammography. Patients who have had a hysterectomy can have varying strengths of oestrogen replacement therapy as tablets, patches or transdermal gel (see *MIMS* for list of HRT preparations and costs). Women who still have a uterus must also take progestogens for part of the month to oppose the proliferation of the endometrium, which could lead to endometrial cancer. Some women who object to having a monthly bleed may prefer a continuous combined HRT but this is contraindicated until at least one year after the last menstrual period.

Sequential combined HRT

The oestrogen tablets, patches or gel are used alone for the first part of the month, and in combination with the progestogen for the latter part. The preparations are used continuously without a break and a bleed usually occurs in the last week of each course. Transdermal patches release quantities of hormone through the skin to maintain the pre-menopausal blood levels. The patch is applied below the waist to the abdomen, buttock or upper thigh and left in place for 3–4 days. It should then be changed, using a fresh patch on a different site. Some patients may experience skin irritation from the adhesive. Patches must not be applied to the breasts. The progestogens may be in tablet form or other patches. Progestogens can produce unwanted side effects such as weight gain, bloating or mood changes and patients may be tempted to skip them unless they understand their importance.

Continuous combined HRT

Continuous combined preparations contain oestrogen and progestogen together to prevent proliferation of the endometrium and thus obviate the need for a monthly bleed. The tablets are taken every day and patients should be warned that some may experience some spotting when first starting the treatment. Combined patches are also available. Tibolone is a synthetic steroid used to control menopausal symptoms and prevent osteoporosis. It can also be helpful for patients with decreased libido.

Slow release hormone implants can be introduced into the abdominal wall through a trochar. Implants need to be renewed about every six months, but some patients can experience menopausal symptoms while their blood levels of oestrogen are still high. Patients who have not had a hysterectomy need to have progestogens as well, for the reasons stated above.

HRT does not act as a contraceptive and peri-menopausal women need to be aware that they could still be fertile. A barrier method or alternative form of contraception may be needed. HRT injections are not available in the UK but sometimes patients may bring them from other countries and request their administration. In such cases, authorisation for administration should be obtained in writing from the GP.

Osteoporosis

Lack of oestrogen affects the density of bone with the consequent risk of fractures of the hip, wrist and spine in later life. The prevention of falls and subsequent fractures is one of the standards in the *National Service Framework for Older People*[19]. Early menopause or a history of infrequent periods are particular risk factors but up to one in three women may develop osteoporosis in their lifetime. However, this is not exclusively a female problem because one in twelve men may also develop the condition[20]. Osteoporosis in men may be linked to low testosterone levels. Other factors known to contribute to osteoporosis include:

- Heavy smoking
- Long-term corticosteroid use
- High alcohol intake
- Physical inactivity
- Malnutrition
- Family history of osteoporosis.

The major problem arises from the loss of the protein matrix of the bone, although a reasonable calcium intake also helps to preserve the bone mass. Patients should understand the importance of a healthy lifestyle. Regular weight-bearing exercise, e.g. walking or dancing, and exposure to sunlight for vitamin D synthesis, can help to delay osteoporosis. Some hospitals undertake bone densitometry to identify the risk of osteoporosis developing. Women at high risk should be encouraged to use hormone replacement therapy for up to ten years to delay the onset of osteoporosis[21]. The slight increase in the risk of breast cancer with long-term use should be weighed against the risk of osteoporosis. The National Osteoporosis Society campaigns to raise awareness of the problem, funds research, and provides advice and support for sufferers.

Treatment

Treatment for osteoporosis includes:

- Analgesia for pain
- Physiotherapy to achieve maximum mobility and prevent falls: weight-bearing exercise can help to maintain bone density
- Hip protectors if at risk from falls and hip fracture
- HRT, tibolone or selective oestrogen receptor modulators (Raloxefene)
- Biphosphonate drugs (alendronate, etidronate and residronate) inhibit bone resorption and increase bone mass
- Calcium and vitamin D supplementation, if dietary intake is insufficient
- Calcitonin – to regulate bone turnover.

Fractures due to osteoporosis cost the NHS billions of pounds every year as well as causing pain and suffering to countless people. Practice nurses are well placed to educate patients about the risks and to encourage them to adopt preventive measures or seek help if needed.

Bladder problems

Women of all ages may experience problems with the urinary bladder. The start of sexual activity or the atrophic changes after the menopause can both contribute to cystitis (see Chapter 8).

Incontinence of urine

The control of bladder function depends on:

- Intact neurological pathways
- Competent pelvic muscles
- The ability to get to the toilet in time.

Childbirth, obesity, lack of exercise and pelvic surgery can all weaken the muscles of the pelvic floor. Chronic constipation can create pressure on the bladder, and diuretics pose a particular problem for elderly people when their mobility is restricted. An assessment of the patient should include an MSU to exclude an infection, testing for diabetes, and a full history, to identify the factors contributing to incontinence. Urodynamic studies may be arranged for patients with severe problems.

Management of urinary incontinence

The GP or practice nurse can make referrals as appropriate to the district nurse, physiotherapist, occupational therapist or local continence adviser. Prime consideration should be given to helping incontinent patients to preserve their dignity. Adaptation of the patient's clothing or the home may make access to the toilet easier for people with reduced mobility or urgency. Patients with dementia may need to be taken to the toilet and encouraged to pass urine at regular intervals. Impacted faeces can cause retention of urine with overflow. Treatment of the underlying problem may relieve the urinary symptoms.

Stress incontinence   This occurs when the abdominal pressure is raised, as in coughing, sneezing or laughing, and the urethral sphincter muscles are unable to prevent the leakage of urine. The degree of urine loss can vary. Treatments include regaining a normal weight and regular pelvic floor exercises. The exercises involve tightening the muscles around the anus as if trying to avoid passing wind, and around the urethra is if trying to stop the stream of urine. Instruction leaflets can be obtained from the health promotion department, or from the Continence Foundation. The physiotherapist may be asked to ensure that the patient understands how to perform pelvic floor exercises, or to improve pelvic muscle tone by electrical stimulation. Patients can obtain special cone-shaped weights to insert into the vagina; muscle tone is improved through the effort needed to keep the cone *in situ*. Cones of a heavier weight can be used as the muscle tone increases. Surgery may be needed to treat severe stress incontinence.

Urge incontinence   This occurs when the patient feels an overwhelming need to pass urine before the bladder is full, and is unable to get to the toilet in time. The bladder muscle starts to contract too soon (detrusor instability). Treatments include:

- Local or systemic oestrogen replacement therapy may help with atrophic changes in older women
- The substitution of drinks containing caffeine such as tea, coffee and cola with plain water may reduce bladder irritability
- Bladder training programmes involving learning to ignore the urge to pass urine for longer and longer periods of time until control of bladder function is regained
- Oxybutynin or tolterodine tartrate may be prescribed to control unstable detrusor contractions.

Some patients may have a combination of stress and urge incontinence. Patients with neurological disorders can also have problems with bladder function and some patients may be taught to empty their bladders by intermittent self-catheterisation. Such teaching is usually done by a specialist continence adviser or a district nurse. Indwelling catheters are avoided as much as possible in the management of bladder problems because of the risk of infection but they are still used at times in the community.

Community trusts will have their own procedures for the assessment and supply of incontinence products for patients who need them. The Department of Health has issued guidelines on the provision of continence care[22]. Urinary incontinence can pose specific problems for women from some minority ethnic groups. The ability to perform ritual cleansing before prayers has been shown to be seriously affected by incontinence, with detrimental effects on the self-esteem and marital relationships of some Muslim women[23]. Practice nurses should be aware that patients who have any communication difficulties, either through language or speech problems, may need help to express their concerns and to receive the service they need.

Information for patients

Leaflets and fact sheets are available on a wide range of topics, but patients may be too embarrassed to pick some of them up in a public waiting area. Careful attention should be given to siting potentially embarrassing information about continence services, family planning, or genito-urinary medicine clinics in appropriate places. People with access to the Internet may prefer to get information that way.

Suggestions for reflection on practice

Consider your service for women in your practice.

- Are any improvements needed to the facilities, equipment or information material?
- Do you need to increase or update any of your knowledge or skills in order to provide a comprehensive service?
- How do you know whether patients are satisfied with the service provided?

Further reading

Andrews, G. (ed.) (1997) *Women's Health*. Bailliere Tindall, London.
Austoker, J. & Davey, C. (1997) *Cervical Smear Results Explained: a guide for primary care*. Cancer Research Campaign, London.
O'Rourke, A. & Roberts, C. (1998) *Cervical Cytology Screening – the problems*. WISDOM Project. *www.shef.ac.uk/uni/projects/wrp/cervical* (accessed 16/10/01).

References

1. Hurskainen, R., Teperi, J., Rissanen, P., *et al.* (2001) Quality of life and cost-effectiveness of levonorgestrel-releasing intrauterine system versus hysterectomy for treatment of menorrhagia: a randomised trial. *Lancet*, **357** (9525), 273–7.
2. National Association for Premenstrual Syndrome (2001) Treatment guidelines for premenstrual syndrome. *Guidelines*, **14**, 224–5.
3. Wyatt, K., Dimmock, P. and O'Brien, P. (2000) Premenstrual syndrome. *Clinical Evidence*, **3**, 942–54.
4. Wyatt, K., Dimmock, P. and O'Brien (2000) Premenstrual syndrome. *Clinical Evidence*, **3**, 942–54.
5. Department of Health (1999) *Saving Lives: Our Healthier Nation*. Department of Health, London.
6. Edwards, M. (2001) Cervical neoplasia. *Practice Nurse*, **22** (1), 23–8.
7. Royal College of Nursing (1995) Bimanual pelvic examination guidance for nurses. *Issues in Nursing and Health*, **34**. Royal College of Nursing, London.
8. Department of Health (2000) *The NHS Cancer Plan*. *www.doh.gov.uk/cancer/cancerplan.htm*

9. CMO and CNO (1998) *Clinical Examination of the Breast*. PL/CNO.98/1, Department of Health, London.
10. Brickner, L., Crowley, P., Neilson, J. & O'Dowd, T. (2000) Antenatal care in low risk pregnancies. *Clinical Evidence*, **3**, 637–8.
11. Great Britain, Parliament (1990) *Human Fertilisation and Embryology Act, 1990*. HMSO, London.
12. BBC News (2001) IVF twin threat questioned. Fertility Conference 2001. *www.bbc.co.uk/hi/english/in_depth/2001/fertilty_conference_2001/newsid_141* (accessed 16/10/01).
13. British Medical Association and the Royal Pharmaceutical Society of Great Britain (2001) *British National Formulary*, **41**, 9.6.1.
14. Simpson, L. (2000) Stress incontinence in younger women: prevention and treatment. *Nursing Standard*, **14** (36), 49–54.
15. Crowther, C. & Middleton, P. (2001) Anti-D administration after childbirth for preventing Rhesus alloimmunisation (Cochrane Review). *The Cochrane Library*, Issue 3. Update Software. *www.update-software.com*
16. Kohner, N. (1995) *Pregnancy Loss and the Death of a Baby: Guidelines for Professionals*. Stillbirth and Neonatal Death Society, London.
17. Amen, F. (undated) Hysterectomy and ovarian preservation. *Stethoscope*. *www.hadbai.co.uk/hysterectomty/* (accessed 17/10/01).
18. Mahavani, V. & Sood, A. (2001) Hormone replacement therapy and cancer risk. *Current Opinions in Oncology*, **13** (5), 384–9.
19. Department of Health (2001) *National Service Framework for Older People*. Department of Health, London.
20. National Osteoporosis Society. *Oseoporosis – The Silent Epidemic. www.nos.org.uk/gener* (accessed 17/8/01).
21. Royal College of Physicians (1999) *Osteoporosis: clinical guidelines for prevention and treatment*. Royal College of Physicians, London.
22. Department of Health (2000) *Good Practice in Continence Services*. Department of Health, London.
23. Wilkinson, K. (2001) Pakistani women's perceptions and experience of incontinence. *Nursing Standard*, **16** (5), 33–9.

Useful addresses and web sites

Cancer BACUP – cancer information service
Web site: *www.cancerbacup.org.uk/*

Issue (The National Fertility Association) formerly the National Association for the Childless
114 Lichfield Street, Walsall, West Midlands
Web site: *www.issue.co.uk/*

Stillbirth and Neonatal Death Society
28 Portland Place, London W1N 4DE
Telephone: 020 7436 5881
Web site: *www.uk.sands.org/*

Web sites

British Menopause Society
Web site: *www.the-bms.org*

National Osteoporosis Society
Web site: *www.nos.org.uk*

The Hysterectomy Association – support group for patients
Web site: *www.hysterectomy association.org.uk/*

Chapter 14
Men's Health

The specific health needs of women have been recognised for many years, and well-woman clinics and screening programmes developed. Men's health has generally received much less attention, although there are several valid reasons for targeting men's health issues.

Morbidity and mortality

The life expectancy of men is, on average, between five and seven years lower than that for women; a fact which is compounded by differences between social classes. Life expectancy in the 1990s for men in professional and managerial jobs was 76 years, while it was only 71 years for men in unskilled or semi-skilled work[1].

Men are four times more likely than women to:

- Commit suicide
- Die from an accident
- Develop heart disease.

Men are also more likely, in general, to die from strokes, cancer or respiratory diseases[2]. Most of the above conditions are included in the targets for reducing mortality in *Saving Lives: Our Healthier Nation*[3].

Suicide

The incidence of depression in men may be equal to that in women, but may not be so recognisable. Women are more likely to seek help from primary care. However, men with depression may resort to other means, and some may mask their distress by violent behaviour or alcohol abuse. The traditional idea of masculinity requires men to be strong, so that accepting help can make them feel unmanly. Boys learn at an early age not to cry or show emotion.

Between 1994 and 1996, 25% of deaths of men in their twenties were due to suicide[4]. Various factors are thought to contribute to the incidence of suicide in men:

- Unemployment – particularly when unemployment carries a greater social stigma[5]
- Older men – possibly due to social isolation, loss of a partner or hopelessness
- Mental illness
- Prisoners (especially those on remand). Criminal activity may also be linked to under-achievement at school, lack of parenting and suitable role models, drug or alcohol abuse, violence
- Farmers – especially during crises in the rural economy
- Occupational groups (doctors, dentists, veterinary surgeons, pharmacists) – may reflect greater knowledge and access to drugs for suicide.

The assessment of the risk for suicide is fraught with difficulty, but practice nurses who are alert to the possibility and who are able to establish a rapport with patients, may be able to identify some warning signs when talking to them. Has the patient:

- Recently felt depressed?
- Been uncharacteristically religious?
- Made a will or been unusually extravagant?
- Talked of self-harm or made plans to self-harm?
- Been unusually elated? (can occur once the decision to end it all has been reached).

Gentle questioning about how the patient sees the future can lead to more direct questions about suicidal intent[6].

The needs of the family and those close to patients who commit suicide, also need consideration. Guilt, anger and depression are all part of the grieving process, but financial problems or behaviour problems in children can also occur. Whatever the situation, it would be useful to know how to help patients who need support, or where to refer them.

Accidents

Some men are socialised to engage in high-risk activities. Even though the value of exercise is strongly promoted, sports injuries are common, ranging from musculo-skeletal injuries, to permanent disability or death. Contact sports carry a risk of serious injury. The desire to impress others, or the adrenaline rush from extreme sports, can lead men in particular, to place their lives in danger. Motorbike and car accidents through reckless driving, are sadly all too common.

Occupational hazards

Despite moves towards sex equality, men are still generally exposed to greater health hazards at work. Men have traditionally been employed in heavy industry, with its attendant risks of accidents. Work-related health problems also include:

- Occupational asthma, from working with dust or fumes.
- Dermatitis, from allergy to chemicals or substances in the work-place.
- Cancer linked to the work environment, e.g. mesothelioma from asbestos.
- Skin cancers from prolonged exposure to the sun.
- Stress – long working hours and the competitive nature of some jobs, combined with the ever-present fear of redundancy, can be detrimental to mental health.
- Post-traumatic stress disorder (see Chapter 15). Some occupations such as the fire brigade, police and ambulance services expose employees to horrifying experiences. Although not the exclusive province of men, women in such occupations may be more able to use the support offered and to express their feelings and show emotion. Men, however, may feel unable to use the counselling services provided for fear of being thought weak or unable to cope.

Health and safety regulations are designed to minimise work-related injuries but some men choose to flout the regulations so as to appear macho. Giving information or providing protective clothing may not be enough – the whole culture may need to be changed. Lunch-time drinking is no longer considered acceptable in many companies, and failure to wear the protective clothing provided is a dismissible offence on some building sites.

Coronary heart disease
(see Chapter 9, Health promotion and Chapter 16, Supporting patients with chronic diseases)

Men have always been known to have a greater incidence of heart disease than women. Oestrogen protects women until the menopause. Then the risk increases; especially in women with a history of smoking. In 1997 it was predicted that one in four men would have a heart attack[7]. The National Service Framework for Coronary Heart Disease sets national standards of care for preventing and treating CHD. Practice nurses are at the forefront of the efforts to meet the standards set for primary care. That is why an understanding of the different ways men view health issues is essential so that different approaches can be tried.

Male patients in general practice

Education for practice nurses on issues of men's health is usually patchy, with specific topics such as sexual health or testicular self-examination being covered in different courses. One important fact to remember is that men are not all alike and any discussion of men's health must consider these differences:

- *Social background and employment*   There may be differences in attitude to health issues in relation to education and social class. The effect of unemployment on physical and mental health is well known. There may be role reversal, with men responsible for childcare while women go out to work. *New man* is the term coined to describe men with a supposedly more progressive attitude to masculinity and femininity[8].

- *Relationships*   Men may have come from homes without a male role model or have been subjected to physical or mental abuse. Such men may have difficulty in making satisfactory relationships. Perpetrators of domestic violence can come from any social class, but those from the higher social classes may not be recognised as being violent. While some men can be the victims of violence by women, it should not be forgotten that most domestic violence is perpetrated by men[9].

- *Cultural background*   Men from different ethnic backgrounds may have particular health risks but be reluctant to attend for a health check. The practice profile should help to identify the specific health risks of men in the local population.

- *Sexual orientation*   Gay men in general may be more aware of their own health needs and have a support network to contact, but younger gay men may still need advice and information. The statistics for HIV and STD infections over time, partly reflect the way the message about safe sex is, or is not, getting through to young men of all sexual persuasions[10]. Male rape of straight or gay men has been in the news in recent years. In a survey published in 1999, 3% of men in England were shown to have been the victims of sexual assault[11]. Although still relatively rare compared to the rape of females, the effect on some men can be totally devastating and victims will need referral for specialised help and support.

- *Disability*   The concept of masculinity and male dominance may be challenged by any form of disability which results in dependence on others.

- *Knowledge*   Some men are ignorant about how their bodies work and what contributes to good health. They may be amenable to information about ways of increasing their fitness. Other men may have a good knowledge of physiology and may, or may not, take care of their health.

Valuing diversity entails accepting people as they are and tailoring the nursing approach to suit their needs.

Women generally have more contact with general practice than men do – especially young men. There could be several reasons why women feel more comfortable in the practice setting:

- A higher proportion of the staff are usually female – receptionists, nurses and often, doctors
- Women are accustomed to personal consultations for contraception, well-woman screening, pregnancy or HRT, or consultations for their children with childhood illnesses or for immunisations.

Surgery times could also deter men from attending well-man clinics because they are unwilling to take time off work when they are not ill. Some men equate visiting the doctor with being sick and they may feel anxious about being amongst ill people. They may have had a bad experience in the past and wish to avoid being told off about their eating, drinking or smoking habits. Moreover, when men do have something wrong with them, they may put off seeing the doctor for a longer period[12].

Traditionally there has been less investment in men's health. The RCN Men's Health Forum reports that for every pound spent on men's health, eight pounds are spent on women[13]. This inequality needs to be addressed and a new approach adopted to health services for men. Enlightened individuals have shown how this can be done. The Health of Man Group (HOM) founded in Bradford and Airedale in 1997 runs drop-in centres for men of all ages[14]. Another innovation by Jane Deville-Almond is the organisation of mobile clinics in places where men gather, such as the pub, and MOT checks for men at the motorbike shop[15]. The nursing journals publish details of these and other ventures; often their success depends on the skills and efforts of charismatic leaders, with good management support. Yet it is hoped that by learning from their successes and setbacks, primary care staff in other areas will be inspired to adopt similar methods. Primary care trusts can incorporate schemes for improving men's health in their health improvement programmes.

Well-man checks

Given the constraints mentioned above, some men will come to see the practice nurse for a new-patient health check (see Chapter 9, Health Promotion). Others may request a general check-up. This may be triggered by a landmark birthday, ill health in a family member or work colleague, or by pressure from a partner. It is always worth finding out what prompted the patient to attend, in order to elicit any particular health concerns. Younger men are more likely to attend for travel advice and immunisations. There would not usually be enough time in a consultation to discuss many general health issues, but safer sex, the risk of accidents and sunburn, especially when associated with alcohol excess, should be included.

In older men there is an increased risk of osteoporosis, as discussed in Chapter 13, Women's Health. The treatment for men may include testosterone, but other aspects will be the same as those for women, listed under Treatment.

Sexual health (see Chapter 12)

Sexual risk-taking is common amongst young men. Peer pressure and the need to save face exert significant influence. Yet many of them do not perceive themselves as having access to the sexual health services available to young women. Young male patients will be unlikely to attend the surgery to discuss their concerns unless they can be guaranteed confidentiality and ease of access[16]. Yet there is a great need for services for this group of patients and some practice nurses feel confident enough to provide such a service. Alternatively, there should be easily accessible information about services in the local area, discretely placed for young people to pick up.

Testicular cancer

Cancer of the testes occurs most commonly in men aged between 20 and 40 years. About 1500 men are affected annually in the UK[15]. The condition is rare in non-Caucasian men. The incidence of testicular cancer has doubled since the 1970s but early detection allows a 90% cure rate. Hence the need for men to be aware of the disease and for them to know how to examine their testicles. Just as women are taught breast awareness, so men need to know how to perform testicular self-examination. Leaflets can be obtained from health promotion departments to back up this education. The earlier the disease is detected and treated, the better the chance of a cure.

Many sexual health courses include testicular self-examination (TSE) in their curricula. Men should be taught to be familiar with the normal weight, texture and consistency of their testes and to examine themselves regularly after a warm bath or shower, when the scrotum is relaxed. The epididymus could be mistaken for a lump if the patient is not aware of the normal anatomy of the testes. It is normal for the testicles to be different in size and for one to be lower than the other[16]. The cause of testicular cancer is not fully understood but factors known to be associated with the condition include undescended testicles, inguinal hernia, and a genetic fault on the maternal X chromosome. Other possible causes under investigation include: testicular torsion, environmental exposure to oestrogen, mumps orchitis, and lack of exercise[17].

Treatment

Removal of the diseased testicle is usually performed. If the remaining testicle is healthy, the patient may still be able to father children, but when fertility is at risk, semen can be collected and frozen for future use. Radiotherapy and chemotherapy may be used post-surgery depending on the type of tumour. The prognosis is usually very good for men without metastatic disease.

The diagnosis of testicular cancer can have a devastating effect on the self-esteem and body image of the men affected. Patients can benefit from a self-help group for men with the same condition. Nurses can provide information about any local group, or encourage the setting up of a group if none exists[18].

Testicular cancer usually affects young men and thus each case can be particularly poignant, despite the relatively small number of cases nationally each year. Information about the importance of TSE can be given to mothers, girlfriends and partners when they attend for well-woman screening, so that they can pass the message on to their menfolk.

Prostate disease

Benign prostatic hyperplasia (BPH)

BPH is a common disease of men over 50 years of age, which if left untreated can lead to recurrent bladder infections, bladder calculi and acute urinary retention[19]. The prostate gland, which is the shape and size of a chestnut, is situated around the urethra at the neck of the bladder. Enlargement of the prostate gland happens gradually, so symptoms tend to develop slowly and patients may accept them as part of the ageing process. Typically there may be:

- Hesitancy – difficulty or delay in starting micturition
- A poor or intermittent urinary stream
- A feeling of not completely emptying the bladder.
- Terminal dribbling
- Nocturia.

All of these symptoms can affect the quality of life of men with BPH. Renal function can be adversely affected and acute retention of urine, apart from causing extreme discomfort, can necessitate surgical removal of the prostate.

Opportunistic questioning during new-patient, well-man and over-75 health checks can help in identifying patients with prostatic symptoms. Ask such questions as:

- Do you have any trouble passing urine?
- Do you have to get up at night to pass water?

If the answer to either of the questions is 'yes', further enquiry may elicit the extent of the problem and the effect on the patient's quality of life. Patients with urinary symptoms should be offered an assessment and examination to rule out prostate cancer and to identify ways of relieving the symptoms. A detailed history is necessary, covering these points:

- An account of any symptoms
- Usual daily fluid intake
- Medication (including diuretics)
- Bowel habit (constipation can cause or exacerbate urinary obstruction)
- Any history of urinary infections or surgery to the urinary tract.

Investigations

Urinalysis is necessary to identify any infection, haematuria or glycosuria. A specimen may be sent for microscopy and culture if an infection is suspected. A blood glucose test may be needed if diabetes is a possibility. A blood test for serum creatinine, will determine if the renal function is impaired. The test for prostate-specific antigen (PSA) is also likely to be requested, but this test can be raised with BPH as well as prostate cancer, so can cause difficulties with interpretation of the result. Digital rectal examination is usually performed by a GP but some nurses are specially trained to undertake the examination. The patient may also be referred for a transrectal ultrasound examination.

Treatment

The following can be used:

- *Watchful waiting*   Men with mild to moderate symptoms, which cause them little inconvenience, may opt to delay treatment. They should be monitored annually.

- *Drug treatment*   This may be offered. Alpha-blockers, e.g. alfuzosin, tamsulosin and terazosin, relax smooth muscle and so may improve urinary flow. These drugs can also cause hypotension so careful monitoring of the blood pressure is necessary. Alpha-blockers are contraindicated for patients who have a history of orthostatic hypotension or micturition syncope[20]. Antiandrogens, e.g. finasteride, inhibit testosterone metabolism, leading to a reduction in prostate size, with subsequent improvement in urinary flow. They are most suitable for men with a prostate volume of more than 40 ml. Decreased libido, erectile dysfunction and ejaculation disorders are some of the possible side effects of finasteride (see *BNF*). Men taking these tablets are advised to use a condom when having sexual intercourse and women who are pregnant or could become pregnant should not handle the tablets if they are crushed or broken.

- *Surgical treatments*   These are more effective in relieving symptoms but have a higher rate of complications such as retrograde ejaculation, erectile dysfunction and urinary incontinence[21].

Prostate cancer

Almost 10 000 men died from prostate cancer in the UK in 1998, making it one of the most common cancers in men[22]. The condition is more common in men over the age of 50 and the risk of developing it rises with age. Half of all prostate cancers occur in men over 75 years of age. The symptoms can be similar to those of BPH, although some men may be asymptomatic, or else present with haematuria.

Apart from age, other risk factors for developing prostate cancer include a family history of the disease and possibly, a diet high in fat. Afro-Caribbean men have a higher risk of developing prostate cancer[22]. The increased incidence may partly relate to improved detection rates through PSA tests, digital rectal examination and trans-rectal ultrasound. However, the earlier diagnosis of the disease could result in the patient undergoing many unpleasant investigations and treatments, when the disease might not have caused serious problems or affected the patient's mortality. The debate about PSA testing relates to this dilemma: the challenge for researchers is to devise a test which can differentiate aggressive tumours which require immediate treatment, from those which can be safely managed by watchful waiting.

Prostate-specific antigen

PSA is a glycoprotein produced by the prostate and released into the bloodstream. Raised levels of PSA in a blood sample may indicate the presence of prostate cancer, but the test is not specific for cancer because prostatitis and BPH can also cause the PSA level to be elevated. Patients may request PSA tests in response to media interest in the subject or government pronouncements. *The NHS Cancer Plan* stated that PSA testing to detect prostate cancer will be made available, supported by information about the risks and benefits, to empower men to make their own choices[23]. Patients must be counselled about the implications of the test so that they can make an informed decision. Leaflets will be supplied to all surgeries explaining the benefits and drawbacks of PSA tests[24].

Gleason score

There are several systems around the world used for grading prostate tumours but the one most commonly used in the UK is Gleason grading. This uses a score from 1 to 5, with 1 being the most well-differentiated, through to 5 being the most poorly differentiated tumour.[25] While such knowledge can be empowering and help patients to make decisions about their treatment, it can also engender anxiety when levels rise. Practice nurses should be able to provide information about cancer support groups and helplines for patients who wish to use them[25].

Treatment

The statistics for the long-term survival of men with prostate cancer, unlike those with testicular cancer, does not appear to change significantly whether they are treated or not. Treatment of aggressive tumours is likely to be more successful if the tumour is localised within the capsule of the prostate. Possible treatments include:

- *Radical prostatectomy*   This can reduce the risk of metastases, but apart from the usual dangers of surgery, carries the risk of sexual dysfunction and urinary incontinence.
- *Radiotherapy and interstitial irradiation (brachytherapy)*   This can cause diarrhoea and proctitis as side effects of the treatment, as well as erectile dysfunction.
- *Drug treatments*   Prostate tumours are generally dependent on testosterone. Orchidectomy is the most radical way of reducing testosterone, but as few men are willing to be castrated, this is usually achieved chemically by the use of luteinising hormone releasing hormone antagonists in order to suppress the release of LHRH by the pituitary gland. Practice nurses may be asked to administer these drugs. They are usually prescribed for men with advanced prostate cancer, in a slow-release preparation, either as an injection, e.g. leuprorelin, or as an implant, e.g. goserelin. The drug company which manufactures goserelin will provide training for nurses and a video on the insertion technique. The manufacturers do not recommend the use of local anaesthetic before insertion of the implant, but some doctors and nurses prefer to anaesthetise the skin first. Anaesthetic cream and an occlusive dressing can be prescribed for the patient to apply one hour before coming to the surgery.

The implant technique is not difficult but should not be attempted before training. Follow this procedure:

(1)   Clean the skin with an alcohol swab or povidone iodine to minimise the risk of introducing infection.
(2)   Instil local anaesthetic to the injection site if needed.
(3)   Check that the pellet can be seen in the neck of the syringe and carefully remove the guard from the plunger to avoid accidentally expelling the pellet.
(4)   Pinch up and hold a fold of skin and subcutaneous tissue of the patient's abdomen with the non-dominant hand.
(5)   Insert the needle subcutaneously into the fold of skin and depress the plunger to insert the implant.
(6)   Withdraw the needle, check the insertion site and apply a small sterile dressing.
(7)   Warn the patient that there may be some bruising after the procedure.

The side effects can be troublesome for some men. They include hot flushes, sweating, gynaecomastia and weight gain. The suppression of testosterone also causes loss of libido and erectile dysfunction. Other side effects are listed in the *BNF*. Nurses administering the drugs should enquire about side effects and if the side effects are troublesome for the patient, either refer the patient to the GP or suggest that the patient discusses them with the urologist. Anti-androgen drugs, e.g. cyproterone acetate, flutamide, bicalutamide, may also be used for advanced disease or to prevent an initial worsening of symptoms, known as tumour flare when LHRH antagonists are first used. Bony metastases commonly occur in the spine and can cause severe pain. Adequate analgesia will be needed but sometimes this can be tailed off if the tumours respond to drug treatment or radiotherapy.

Erectile dysfunction (ED)

Erectile dysfunction, previously called impotence, can be described as the persistent inability to obtain or maintain sufficient rigidity of the penis to allow satisfactory sexual activity. The condition is often associated with ageing but should not be dismissed as such until other causes have been ruled out. The portrayal of sex by the media and the pressures on men related to changes in their role in society, can undermine the sexual confidence of many men. The inability to achieve or maintain an erection can affect a man's self-esteem and damage the relationship with a partner. Some men, being unable to discuss the problem, may avoid physical contact altogether, with the result that their partner feels unloved and rejected.

Erectile dysfunction is not a disease; it is a complication of other conditions. Thus the causes of ED may be physical, psychological or a combination of both:

- *Endocrine disorders*   Up to 75% of men with diabetes mellitus may have ED[26]. Testosterone insufficiency, abnormal thyroid function, hyperprolactinaemia and excess growth hormone may all cause ED.

- *Vascular disease*   Arteriosclerosis can affect the blood flow through the penis. Cardiovascular disease and hypertension are associated disorders.

- *Surgery and radiotherapy*   These can cause damage to the cavernous nerves or the pelvic plexus. Altered body image after surgery can also be a psychogenic cause.

- *Drugs*   Both prescribed and illicit drugs may affect erectile function, e.g. antidepressants, antipsychotics, antihypertensives, diuretics, anticholinergics, some hormones, anti-androgens, anticonvulsants, antiparkinson drugs, fibrates, H_2 antagonists and psychotropic drugs including alcohol.

- *Sedentary lifestyle*   Lack of exercise has been shown to be a modifiable risk factor for ED[27].

- *Neurodegenerative disorders*

- *Anatomical deformities of the penis* Peyronie's disease is characterised by fibrosis in the shaft of the penis, which may require surgical correction.

- *Psychogenic causes* Depression, anxiety, stress disorders and psychoses may be primary causes. Performance anxiety and fear of failure or rejection can compound the situation, whatever the primary cause.

Patients would not usually consult the practice nurse primarily to discuss ED, unless the nurse is known to have a specialist qualification in this field of sexual health. However, up to one in ten men experience the problem at some time, so nurses are likely to encounter men with ED in any clinical setting. The possibility should be borne in mind at any health check or consultation for chronic disease management. It may be necessary to explain that many drugs and illnesses are known to have an effect on sexual functioning and that help is available if it is ever needed. Open-ended questions may help some patients to articulate any worries about sexual matters.

Assessment and investigations

A full medical, social and sexual history is needed, together with the patient's view of the problem and that of the sexual partner. It is important to establish how and when the problem started and to understand what happens when the patient anticipates love-making and whether erections occur at night or when waking up. Any medication being taken should be checked for known effects on erectile function. Whether this interview will be carried out by a nurse or a doctor will depend on individual practice circumstances. A patient would quickly sense any embarrassment by the practitioner, with a detrimental effect on the consultation and any future progress. Blood pressure should always be measured and a blood test taken for undiagnosed diabetes. A physical examination should identify any anatomical abnormalities of the penis or testes as well as signs of peripheral vascular or neurological disease. Other blood tests will depend on individual circumstances but could include:

- Full blood count
- Thyroid function, especially if loss of libido
- Hormone profile – testosterone, prolactin, follicle-stimulating hormone and luteinising hormone.

Treatment

Any underlying physical cause should be addressed and any medication reviewed. Alternative drugs may be prescribed in some instances. Psychosexual counselling may be appropriate for some patients and their partners.

Drug treatments

The licensing of sildenafil brought erectile dysfunction into the public arena for a while, when the topic was discussed freely in the press and on prime-time television. Drug treatments for ED may only be prescribed on NHS prescriptions for men with specific medical conditions (see *BNF*). Such prescriptions must be endorsed SLS to be valid. The following drugs may be prescribed:

- Sildenafil (Viagra) 50 or 100 mg tablet taken one hour before expected sexual activity. It is contraindicated for patients taking nitrates because it can potentiate their hypotensive effect, and when vasodilatation or sexual activity is inadvised, because of a recent stroke or myocardial infarction.
- Alprostadil (Prostaglandin E_1) may be given as a tablet inserted by an applicator into the male urethra (MUSE) or by intracavernous injection (Caverject, Virida). A condom should be used if there is any possibility of pregnancy in the partner. Priapism can be a serious side effect and patients should be advised to seek medical help if an erection lasts longer than four hours.
- Yohimbine (not available on prescription) is derived from the bark of the African yohimbine tree. It has been found to be more effective than placebo, without having serious side effects[28]. More trials are needed to compare the effect with other treatments.

Vacuum constriction devices

Various devices are available. Vacuum pumps draw blood into the penis and a constriction ring is then placed over the base of the penis to maintain rigidity. The penis can feel cold because of the restricted blood flow and the constricting ring should not be left on for longer than 30 minutes because of the risk of ischaemia. Patients taking anticoagulants should not use this method, owing to the risk of haemorrhage within the penis.

Prosthesis

As a last resort, some men may have a prosthesis implanted surgically. This can entail destruction of the patient's own cavernous tissue to accommodate the implant. Infection is a serious complication which may occur in 2–7% of cases[29].

Conclusion

Erectile dysfunction is a cause of anxiety and embarrassment to thousands of men. Recognising the problem and knowing where to get information and help is an important first step. Practice nurses are ideally placed to ensure that the health needs of male patients receive equal attention to those of women.

Suggestions for reflection on practice

- How friendly is your surgery towards men?
  - Are appointment times appropriate?
  - Are there magazines for men in the waiting area?
- How well-equipped are you to deal with men's health issues?
  - Could any changes be made?

Further reading

Luck, M., Bamford, M. & Williamson, P. (2000) *Men's Health Perspectives, Diversity and Paradox*. Blackwell Science, Oxford.

Vaughan, A. (2000) Walk-in clinic – erectile dysfunction. *Practice Nursing*, **11** (19), 29–35.

References

1. Office for National Statistics (1999) *Health Statistics Quarterly*, Spring Edition, p. 6.
2. Deville-Almond, J. (2000) Man troubles. *Nursing Times*, **96** (11), 28–29.
3. Department of Health (1999) *Saving Lives: Our Healthier Nation*. Department of Health, London.
4. Office for National Statistics (1999) *Health Statistics Quarterly*, Spring Edition, p. 38.
5. Duffy, D. (2000) Suicide and deliberalte self-harm. In: *Lyttle's Mental Health and Disorder* (eds. T. Thompson and P. Mathias), 3rd edn. pp 390–401. Balliere Tindall, London.
6. Office of National Statistics (1997) *Population Trends*. HMSO, London.
7. Collier, R. (1992/3) The new man: fact or fad. *Achilles Heel*, 14. *www.achillesheel.freeuk.com/achilles14_9*
8. Department of Health (2000) *Domestic Violence: a Resource Manual for Health Care Professionals*. Department of Health Publications, London.
9. Public Health Laboratory Service (2000). *AIDS, HIV Quarterly Surveillance Tables*. PHLS, London.
10. Coxell, A. King, M., Mezey, G. & Gordon, D. (1999) Lifetime prevalence, characteristics and associated problems of non-consensual sex in men: cross sectional survey. *British Medical Journal*, **318** (7187), 846–50.
11. Dirckze, S. (2000) How to persuade men to visit the surgery. *Practice Nurse*, **20** (5), 266–8.
12. Perry, M. (2000) Dead men walking. *Nursing Times*, **96** (11), 29.
13. Chell, S., Jones, D., Hughes, N. & Saunders, R. (2000) Men's health: slugs and snails? *Practice Nursing*, **11** (17), 5–9.
14. Gill, H. (2000) Sexual health is an issue for young men, too. *Practice Nurse*, **20** (5), 270–73.
15. McBride, S. (1998) Below the belt. *Nursing Times*, **94** (22), 29–30.
16. Cook, R. (2000) Teaching and promoting testicular self-examination. *Nursing Standard*, **14** (24), 48–51.

17. Buetow, S. (1995) Epidemiology of testicular cancer. *Epidemiologic Review*, **17** (2), 433–49.
18. Clark, A., Jones, P., Newbold, S., Spencer, J., Wilson, M. & Brandwood, K. (2000) Practice development in cancer care: self-help for men with testicular cancer. *Nursing Standard*, **14** (50), 41–6.
19. Kirby, R. (2000) The natural history of benign prostatic hyperplasia. *Urology*, **56** (5 Suppl 1), 3–6.
20. BNF (2001) *British National Formulary*, **41**, 7.4.1. British Medical Association and Royal Pharmaceutical Society of Great Britain.
21. Anonymous (updated 2000) Benign Prostatic Hyperplasia. *Prodigy Guideline. www.prodigy.nhs.uk* (accessed 24/10/01).
22. Angle, A. (2000) Increasing awareness of men's cancers. *Practice Nursing*, **11** (10), 11–14.
23. Department of Health (2000) Extending cancer screening. *The NHS Cancer Plan*, para. 25. *www.doh.gov.uk/cancer/* (accessed 16/8/01).
24. Donaldson, L. (2001) Informed Choice Project for PSA testing. *CMO's Update*, **31**, 8. Department of Health, London.
25. Prostate Cancer UK (undated) *Understanding Gleason Grading. www.prostatecanceruk/org/gleason* (accessed 25/10/01).
26. Ledda, A. (2000) Diabetes, hypertension and erectile dysfunction. *Current Medical Research Opinion*, **16** (Suppl. 1), S17–20.
27. Derby, C., Mohr, B., Goldstein, I., Feldman, H., Johannes, C. & McKinlay, J. (2000) Modifiable risk factors and erectile dysfunction: can lifestyle factors modify risk? *Urology*, **56** (2), 302–6.
28. O'Leary, M. (2000) Erectile dysfunction. *Clinical Evidence*, **5**, 606.
29. O'Leary, M. (2000) Erectile dysfunction. *Clinical Evidence*, **5**, 611.

Useful addresses and web sites

CancerBACUP
3 Bath Place, Rivington Street, London EC2A 3JR
Telephone: 0171 613 2121
Helpline: 0808 800 1234
Web site: *www.cancerbacup.org.uk*

Men's Health Forum
Tavistock House, Tavistock Square, London WC1H 9QB
Telephone: 020 7388 4449
Web site: *www.menshealthforum.org.uk*

Prostate Cancer Charity
Du Cane Road, London W12 0NN
Telephone: 020 8383 8124
Helpline: 0845 300 8383
Web site: *www.prostate-cancer.org.uk*

SPOD (Association to aid the sexual and personal relationships of people with disability)
288 Camden Road, London N7 0 BJ
Telephone: 020 7607 8851

Web site – information on support groups

www.webhealth.co.uk/Self Help and Support Groups

Chapter 15
Mental Health

Holistic care grew from the recognition that physical, mental, social and spiritual well-being are all closely interlinked[1]. Modern nursing courses place emphasis on caring for the whole person within the community. Mental health nursing has always been a separate specialty, and only a small proportion of practice nurses had been educated as mental health nurses at the time of the last national survey[2]. The pace and competitiveness of modern life means that more people are seeking help for stress-related illnesses; while at the same time, the closure of psychiatric institutions has shifted the focus of mental health care to the community. Just as many adults are likely to have some form of mental illness at any one time as there are people with asthma, according to the foreword to the *National Service Framework for Mental Health*[3]. The NSF specifies the standards expected for adults up to the age of 65. *The National Service Framework for Older People* includes mental health standards for people aged over 65 years. The staff in general practice must be able to contribute to new flexible mental health services.

The historical background to the development of mental health services

In the eighteenth century mentally ill people whose families could not afford to confine them in private madhouses, usually ended up in prison or the work-house. During the nineteenth century the state assumed responsibility for the care of lunatics by building huge county asylums in sparsely populated areas. Social reformers campaigned for a more humane treatment of the inmates.

The asylums continued to expand during the first quarter of the twentieth century but there was also a move towards alternative management. Voluntary patients and outpatients began to be treated. The county asylums came under the control of the regional hospital boards when the NHS was founded, but the provision of after care was in the hands of the local authorities.

The development of phenothiazine drugs in the 1950s and 1960s revolutionised the treatment of patients with schizophrenia and reduced the time they needed to be in hospital. A series of scandals, enquiries and reports brought the services for mentally ill and mentally handicapped people into public focus in the 1960s and 1970s[4,5]. At the same time there was a growth in new care facilities: day centres, hostels, and psychiatric units in general hospitals. Community psychiatric nurses grew in numbers and the first CPN post-registration course began in 1974.

The move towards care in the community led to the National Health Service and Community Care Act (1990). The closure of the Victorian institutions, which had begun in the preceding decades, was not matched by adequate facilities for community care. There were success stories of people rehabilitated after years of confinement, but a huge burden was also placed on many families and carers. The acute psychiatric units in some inner city areas were unable to cope adequately with the demand for acute admissions.

The care programme approach (CPA) was introduced in 1991 with the aim of improving community care services for all people with a mental health problem through:

- An assessment of health and social care needs
- A detailed written care plan
- Appointment of a key-worker
- Regular reviews of the plan and changes as necessary.

The lack of resources to meet this ambitious policy and concerns that the available services would be overstretched, led to only the patients perceived as being vulnerable being selected for the CPA. Health authorities all developed their own criteria for deciding which patients should be selected. The National Health Service had the responsibility for the CPA but care management was the responsibility of social services[6].

A change of government in 1997 resulted in ideas for radical changes to the National Health Service, with the stated intention of modernising the entire organisation. Mental health was accorded a high priority and additional funding was promised[7]. The needs of carers were given prominence and public involvement at all levels began to be encouraged. The NHS Plan promised, among other things, hundreds of mental health teams to provide an immediate respond to crises, patient advocates to be set up in every hospital, and improved primary care in deprived areas[8]. The NSF expressed the Government's intention to bring mental health laws up to date to reflect modern treatments. The care programme approach and care management had already been found to be poorly coordinated; a review of the whole process was undertaken and a policy booklet was published in the year 2000, with the aim of achieving:

- Integration of the CPA and care management
- Consistency of implementation nationally
- A more streamlined process to reduce bureaucracy
- A proper focus on the needs of service users[9].

Systems were required to demonstrate the quality of services provided, with joint auditing processes where different agencies were working together.

Mental health care in general practice

Despite the way the term is used in the NSF, mental health should encompass much more than mental illness. Health promotion is usually equated with physical health, with little attention paid to promoting mental health. Moreover, it should be remembered that people with mental health problems are entitled to expect the same screening and health promotion services as the rest of the population; the physical health needs of people with mental illnesses can easily be overlooked[10]. Conversely, people with physical illnesses have a higher rate of mental health problems than the general population. Depending on his/her previous experience and training, a practice nurse might become involved in some of the ways described below.

The promotion of mental health

Regular sleep, exercise, healthy food, and secure relationships all contribute to physical and mental well-being. Nurses can provide practical help and advice as required on healthy living, and also contribute to local and national initiatives to deter people of all ages from substance abuse.

Grief is a natural process in response to a loss, but it can turn into an abnormal reaction if it is not faced and worked through. Bereavement counselling or support groups may be needed to help a patient to deal with grief successfully. Hospices usually run training programmes for nurses on helping the bereaved. People need a chance to talk about the intense emotional and physical feelings they experience. Sometimes, when a person has died suddenly, the one left behind is burdened by a lot of things left unsaid; or words spoken in haste, which are regretted. Support groups are available in some areas for people bereaved in particular circumstances, such as parents who lose children, or those bereaved through violence or major disasters.

The difficulties of modern living, relationship problems, or being the victim of crime, can all cause their own problems. Recognition and acknowledgement of their existence can be the first step, so that help can be provided before a person's mental health is seriously affected.

The recognition and treatment of mental illness

The mental health NSF lists the people most vulnerable to mental health problems. Standard one requires all health and social services to work with individuals and communities, combat discrimination and promote social inclusion. Nurses working in areas with high unemployment, or in rural communities affected by farming disasters like BSE and foot and mouth disease, may encounter a higher than usual number of people with depressive illnesses. *Saving Lives: Our Healthier Nation* has a target for reducing deaths from suicide by at least a fifth by 2010.

Short-term memory problems can alert the staff to a patient's impaired mental function when he/she telephones repeatedly to ask the same questions. Many patients are aware of their memory loss and become anxious about the future. Depression in older people may be masked by anxiety and impaired memory, but the onset of dementia should also be considered.

Practice nurses may be required to administer regular depot injections to patients with psychotic illnesses. An understanding of the possible side effects of the medication is required (see below). Drug treatments need to be well-monitored. Patients with mental illnesses who request repeat prescriptions inappropriately may be missing medication, taking too much, or stockpiling it. The GP should be informed of any concerns.

Support and care for mentally ill patients and their carers

Carers may be under strain and require more support or help to manage at home. Standard six of the mental health NSF details the rights of carers to have their needs assessed and to agree a written care plan for the person being cared for. The needs of young carers must also be addressed. Staff in general practice are likely to know of children or young people who have a mentally ill relative at home. Standard three of the NSF expects people with common mental health problems to be able to access services at any time of the day or night.

When a patient is well known to a practice, the nurse might recognise when a patient's mood or behaviour has altered. A prompt referral to the GP or the community mental health nurse could prevent a further deterioration. When a crisis does occur, a crisis intervention team from the mental health unit might be able to provide an early intensive input within the patient's home. However, sometimes a patient will need acute admission to hospital. If the patient does not accept voluntary admission, compulsory admission is permitted under the Mental Health Act (1983) if he/she is considered to be a danger to him/herself or others. Serious efforts are made to safeguard the civil liberties of such patients.

The Government intends to reform the existing mental health laws and has issued a white paper outlining the new legal framework[12]. The legislation, which aims to be compatible with the Human Rights Act (1998), includes new safeguards and a right to independent advocacy for patients who need compulsory care or treatment. A three stage process is proposed:

- Stage 1: preliminary examination by two doctors and a social worker or another suitably trained mental health professional to decide whether the patient might be at risk of serious harm or pose a risk to others, without specialist mental health treatment.

- Stage 2: formal assessment and treatment as set out in a formal care plan for up to 28 days. After that time a mental health tribunal must confirm any continuing use of compulsory powers.
- Stage 3: a care and treatment order can be made by a mental health tribunal, authorising the care and treatment specified in the care plan for up to six months for the first two orders and up to twelve months for subsequent orders.

The new legislation is also expected to allow compulsory care and treatment orders for patients in the community but medication will only be allowed to be given forcibly in a clinical setting. Community orders will specify the steps to be taken if a patient does not comply with the order, to prevent the risk of harm to him/herself or others.

Dealing with aggression and violence

People who are aggressive or violent are not necessarily mentally ill, but mental illness can sometimes manifest itself in this way. Patients who are very anxious or who have never learned to control their emotions can become abusive if they have to wait to see a doctor. Others can become violent under the influence of alcohol or drugs. Practice nurses and receptionists may be in the front line. Prevention is better than cure, and the time to consider staff safety is before an incident occurs.

Risk assessment

A survey of the practice layout and work arrangements should reveal anything which makes the staff vulnerable. Safety features should be incorporated in the design of practices and health centres. There must be a way of getting help quickly; as well as a practice policy specifying the action to be taken if an aggressive incident occurs. A member of staff could be at risk while alone in the building. In such instances the front door should be kept locked, and a safety chain put on before opening the door to callers.

Nurses and doctors who undertake home visits need to consider the potential dangers and take appropriate precautions:

- Make sure someone knows where you have gone and when to expect you back. A mobile telephone is essential.
- Get all the relevant details of the patient's history and social situation beforehand.
- Report back after finishing the visits, or if delayed.
- Arrange a coded message to be used if help is needed. All the staff must understand the significance of such a message.
- Be aware of any danger signs such as abusive language, strange behaviour or dangerous weapons on view. Do not enter if in doubt.

- Carry a personal alarm to attract attention if attacked in the street.
- Report any worrying incidents to the GP, and to the police (if appropriate).

All staff should have access to training in ways of dealing with difficult situations. The Suzy Lamplugh Trust, a charity run for that specific purpose, provides guidance, resources and training in all matters of personal safety. Some things to consider for avoiding incidents in the practice:

- *Keep patients informed* of what is happening and offer alternative choices if a delay is inevitable.

- *Listen to what the patient is saying*   Allow frustrations to be expressed, without responding defensively. Acknowledge any legitimate cause for complaint and apologise.

- *Avoid confrontation*   Use a quiet, calm voice even if the patient is shouting. Adopt a non-threatening posture and do not fold the arms, as this can be interpreted as aggression. Avoid staring; this can be interpreted as provocation. Try to get the patient away from others in the vicinity.

- *Get someone to phone for the police* if a situation looks likely to get out of control.

- *Avoid being injured*   Stand just out of arm's reach, with the body at an angle so it is not square-on to the patient. Have one foot slightly in front of the other to allow the body to tilt backwards. Endeavour to have a clear escape route and keep an eye out for anything which the patient might use as a weapon. Politely ask the patient to put down a weapon being held. Look out for something to use as a shield in case it is needed. Don't intervene if the patient breaks something; this can be a way of letting off steam[13].

Reporting incidents

A report should be made of any aggressive incidents. Verbal abuse should be recorded in the patient's records. Any violence, or injuries inflicted must be documented in an incident report, as well as in the records. Staff who have been subjected to aggression require a debriefing session to discuss their feelings about the incident. Professional counselling may be needed in some instances. Analysis of a critical incident will allow people to learn from it.

Helping patients with mental health problems

It is beyond the scope of this book to discuss all the ways mental illness might be manifested. This chapter deals mainly with the situations which practice nurses are most likely to encounter.

Stress

The word *stress* is often used nowadays to indicate any situation in which a person feels unable to cope with life's demands. The problems of chronic habituation to tranquillisers have led to the search for safer ways to help. The distressing symptoms of stress derive from biological reactions which evolved to help our primitive ancestors to survive in the face of danger – the fight or flight response. There is usually a balance within the body between the para-sympathetic and sympathetic nervous activity; but the outpouring of adren-aline in response to perceived danger stimulates the sympathetic nervous system. This is predominantly responsible for the effects associated with stress. At the same time, parasympathetic stimulation of the gastrointestinal tract can also result in nausea and diarrhoea.

A certain level of arousal is needed for normal social functioning, and to avoid accidents. Long periods of understimulation will result in boredom, loss of concentration and apathy. Prolonged overstimulation can cause a break-down in the body's ability to adapt, resulting in physical or mental illness. There may be a genetic link with the way individuals react to stress. Something which might overwhelm one person, could seem an exciting challenge to another. Single major stressors such as bereavement, divorce or business failure may precipitate a stress-related illness; or there may be multiple small events until a crisis point is reached.

Patients can consult the GP or nurse with a variety of symptoms which are ultimately attributed to stress: insomnia, depression, constant tiredness, panic attacks, muscular pains, indigestion, skin disorders, or headaches. Counselling might help a patient to identify the problems, and find an appropriate solution. A situation incapable of a solution is not really a problem – it's a fact of life. Sometimes people need help to differentiate between the two.

Depending on the circumstances, various strategies or support agencies might be appropriate:

- *Developing self-awareness* Helping the individual to understand his/her behaviour; to learn to express powerful feelings, such as anger, grief, fear, or guilt; and to accept the need for other people.

- *Assertiveness training* Learning to express personal needs or to refuse requests without giving offence.

- *Dealing with relationships*
  - Children. The health visitor can often advise on parenting skills, to mini-mise the conflict with children. Childcare arrangements may allow parents some freedom. Referral for family therapy may be needed for disturbed children.
  - Partners. Advice about birth control can help in limiting the size of families. Counselling services such as Relate, or some churches, can help with relationship problems. Gay and lesbian self-help groups can provide

specific support. Bereavement counselling services are available for bereaved partners.

- Dependants. Community nurses and social services can provide help for carers. Respite care may be arranged, and carers' associations can provide practical and emotional help.

- *Finance*   Learning to live within an income, or deal with debts (Citizens Advice Bureaux will advise). Ensuring benefits are being claimed (if applicable). Leaflets about entitlement can be obtained from main post offices and social security offices.

- *Time-management*   Learning to identify priorities for action, and to make time for recreation and rest.

- *Enjoying work*   Learning to delegate, or even looking for alternative work if not happy.

- *Finding alternatives*   Unemployment, retirement, or children leaving home can leave a big gap in a patient's life. Part-time work, voluntary work, a hobby or study might help.

- *Relaxation*   Learning to counteract the physical effects of stress by: physical exercise, yoga, therapeutic massage, aromatherapy, or relaxation exercises and tapes.

Post-traumatic stress disorder has been recognised in recent years as a particular type of stress-related illness. It was originally associated with major incidents like train crashes or fires but is now used to describe the range of psychological symptoms people may experience after any traumatic event, including witnessing or being involved in a car crash, violent crime or assault. The symptoms, which may emerge at any time after the event, include: nightmares, panic attacks, loss of memory and concentration, extreme tiredness, and flashbacks. The value of counselling after such events still has to be proved[14].

Disorders of affect (disturbance of mood)

Depression

Depression is characterised by a low mood which affects the ability to carry out everyday activities. Women are twice as likely to be affected as men. The condition can sometimes be overlooked in a patient who presents with multiple physical symptoms. Other symptoms of depression can include:

- Sleep disturbance, often early-morning wakening and being unable to go back to sleep
- Feeling tired all the time

- Lack of concentration
- Loss of libido
- Agitation or irritability
- Feelings of worthlessness or guilt
- Thoughts of self-harm or suicide.

Possible physical causes for some of the symptoms (anaemia or hypothyroidism) are usually ruled out through blood tests. The diagnosis of depression is made clinically, possibly with the aid of a depression questionnaire, such as the Hospital Anxiety and Depression scale[15] or the Two Question test, 'During the last month, have you often been bothered by feeling down, depressed or hopeless?', 'During the last month, have you often been bothered by little interest or pleasure in doing things?'[16].

The treatment of depression will usually depend on the severity of the condition. Mild to moderate depression will sometimes be helped by talking therapies, but severe depression is more likely to respond to antidepressant drug treatments[17]. St John's Wort available from health food shops, is currently very popular and may be beneficial for treating mild to moderate depression. Patients should be warned that it can interact with other drugs, including the contraceptive pill, anti-epilepsy drugs, digoxin and warfarin[18].

Post-partum affective disorders[19]   These may affect new mothers in the following ways:

- Baby blues affect a large number of new mothers. Emotional lability and tearfulness starts within a week of childbirth and is usually self-limiting, but could progress to depression.
- Post-natal depression is a clinical depression which can affect about one in ten mothers. Health visitors often use a tool such as the Edinburgh Post-natal Depression Scale to help identify mothers with depression, but all primary care team members should be alert to the problem and refer if concerned.
- Puerperal psychosis is an acute psychotic illness, characterised by delusions and confusion, in the immediate post-partum period. Urgent psychiatric treatment is needed.

Bi-polar affective disorder

Patients with this condition, also known as manic depression, experience extreme mood swings between deep depression and wild elation. There may be periods of normality in between. The condition tends to run in families and there may be a genetic link[20].

Mania

The patient is over-energetic and enthusiastic, with rapid speech and thought processes. Grandiose schemes, flights of fancy, and wild financial expenditure can cause great distress to the families affected. Sometimes the mania alternates with bouts of black depression, with periods of normality in between.

Treatment of mania   Antipsychotic drugs may be prescribed. Lithium carbonate is commonly used to control the mood swings. Blood levels need to be taken regularly to maintain a therapeutic dose and avoid toxicity. The blood sample should be obtained just before the next dose is due, so the residual blood level is established. The time elapsed since the last dose should be recorded on the pathology request form.

Psychotic disorders

Patients with psychotic disorders have a different way of viewing themselves and the world. Their behaviour may endanger themselves and cause distress or fear to others. Help is then needed to prevent injury and restore the patient's ability to function within society. The disordered thought processes and behaviour can be manifested in many ways.

Schizophrenia

Schizophrenia is a chronic illness characterised by disordered perceptions of reality. The speech pattern may be bizarre; emotions may either be dulled or wholly inappropriate to the situation; the person may be withdrawn or self-absorbed, or behave in ways which seem incongruous in their context; normal tasks cannot be completed. Hallucinations may affect any of the senses, but are most commonly auditory. There may be delusions of persecution, or of grandeur. Patients with paranoid delusions may have bizarre ideas that neighbours are sending magnetic rays into their home or that they are receiving special messages through their television set. Delusions of grandeur may make the patient think that he or she is a famous personage. Patients with schizophrenia have a higher risk of committing suicide[21].

Treatment   Antipsychotic drugs are given to relieve the symptoms of schizophrenia. The choice of drug is usually made by a psychiatrist. They may be oral or parenteral preparations. The main side effect is Parkinsonism because antipsychotic drugs are thought to work by blocking dopamine receptors in the brain. Restlessness, abnormal face and body movements, intention tremor and muscle rigidity are Parkinsonian symptoms; some of which may be mistaken for symptoms of schizophrenia. Patients with extrapyramidal symptoms are usually given anticholinergic drugs, e.g. procyclidine, to counteract the symptoms (see *BNF*). These drugs can, in turn, cause a dry mouth or gastro-intestinal disturbance. They are also liable to abuse and can cause excitement, mental disturbance or confusion, especially in high doses.

    Clozapine can cause agranulocytosis, so monitoring of the white cell count is a condition of the product licence. Regular blood samples are sent by post or courier to the Clozaril Patient Monitoring Service. All the equipment and postage material is supplied by the CPMS. Practice nurses who administer depot neuroleptic injections, e.g. flupenthixol (Depixol), haloperidol decanoate (Haldol), fluphenazine (Modecate), zuclopenthixol (Clopixol), should be aware of the following points and seek advice if necessary:

- *Authorisation* There must be a written prescription signed by the GP or hospital psychiatrist for each patient. The dose may need to be adjusted periodically, and it is important that the nurse is aware of any changes.

- *Stocks* Drugs for injection can either be obtained by each patient on individual prescriptions; or be purchased by the practice and reimbursement claimed for personally administered items.

- *Administration* Depot injections should be administered by deep IM injection using a Z-track method. They should not be given if a patient is pregnant.

- *Side effects* At each visit the patient should be asked how the injection is helping and if it is causing any problems. Some patients gain weight with the medication or develop Parkinsonian side effects.

- *Records* The injections given must be documented appropriately.

- *Monitoring* Annual blood tests for urea and electrolytes and liver function tests may be needed to detect any dysfunction.

The time intervals between injections can vary from weekly to monthly, according to the patient's needs. The patient should be encouraged to make the next appointment before leaving. Reminders may have to be arranged for patients who forget to attend.

Dementia

Dementia is a group of symptoms caused by a number of conditions which affect the brain. Loss of memory for recent events is an early sign of dementia. An inability to perform everyday tasks or to interact socially can follow, as all the higher mental functions become impaired. The degree and speed of impairment can vary between patients. The diagnosis is made clinically, once all the other causes of confusion have been eliminated. Computerised tomography or magnetic resonance imaging can also be used.

Looking after a person with dementia can pose enormous strains on the caregivers. Practice nurses can offer a friendly ear as well as ensuring that carers receive information about all the services, benefits and support available. Many local authorities and voluntary services produce a directory of local services. The Alzheimer's Disease Society provides information and practical support. Many of the volunteers have had personal experiences of caring for a relative with dementia. There are also support groups for people with other sorts of dementia, for example, Parkinson's disease, Huntingdon's chorea, or AIDS.

A balance needs to be maintained between helping people with dementia as their faculties decline, and making them unnecessarily dependent. Carers need help to identify realistic expectations and to take some risks.

Variant Creutzfeldt-Jakob disease (vCJD) is a brain disease, which could affect many more people in the future. The symptoms of the early stages of the disease may be mistaken for other psychiatric conditions, such as depression, anxiety, panic attacks, delusions, paranoia or hallucinations. Other neurological symptoms soon develop, for example, forgetfulness, clumsiness and loss of balance, progressing to dementia, and increasing immobility and helplessness[22]. An urgent search for a cure is underway but more people could be seen with this distressing condition in general practice in the years to come. Young people are often affected, with devastating consequences for their families.

Substance abuse

Drugs have been used for their mind-altering properties for millennia. Taxes on tobacco and alcohol provide the Inland Revenue with vast sums of money every year, and drug dealing is the only growth industry in some inner city areas. Dependence on an addictive substance occurs when a person cannot cope without it. Physical or psychological dependence eventually causes the body to develop tolerance to the substance and ever larger amounts are needed to create the same effect. Severe physical or psychological withdrawal effects are experienced if the substance is not available for any reason.

Alcohol

Alcohol in small quantities is not usually harmful, and there may even be some beneficial effects[23]. Alcohol is a central nervous system depressant, although initially it may create a sense of euphoria. Situations as diverse as accidents, suicide, hypertension and teenage pregnancy can often be linked to the abuse of alcohol. Regular alcohol use can result in dependence. Deprivation of alcohol can then cause depression, anxiety, convulsions and terrifying hallucinations. Practice nurses may identify patients who already have or are in danger of developing a dependence on alcohol and provide help or refer for specialist advice (see Chapter 9, Health Promotion).

Patients who seek help for alcohol dependence may be referred for detoxification. Long-term support will be needed to cope afterwards. Alcoholics Anonymous and other self-help groups provide peer support. Al-Anon and Al-Ateen provide support for the families of problem drinkers.

The use of drugs and other substances depends to a certain extent on both their availability and on social pressures. Now that smoking is less socially acceptable to many people, smokers may find themselves outnumbered at social gatherings. On the other hand, the peer pressure to experiment can be hard for young people to resist and alcohol, tobacco, drugs and solvents are readily available. Illicit drugs have a large number of street names. Information about drugs and their effects can be obtained from the Internet or from the local drug dependency unit.

Opiates

Heroin is an opium derivative with powerful analgesic properties which can also induce a sense of euphoria. The drug may be injected, smoked or inhaled. Tolerance quickly develops, so larger quantities are required. Self-neglect, weight loss, anaemia and infections can follow. The absence of quality control with illegal drugs means that they often contain impurities. However, accidental overdosing with unusually pure forms can result in death. Abscesses and septicaemia can develop from dirty needles, and users who share equipment or who prostitute themselves to get money for drugs, are at risk of developing and spreading HIV infection and hepatitis.

Cocaine is a powerful stimulant derived from the coca plant, which creates a psychological dependence. It is usually sniffed or smoked. Crack, a highly addictive concentrated form of cocaine is readily available and posing a problem for the law enforcement agencies.

Amphetamines

Amphetamines are stimulants which create a feeling of increased energy and excitement. The user is restless and overactive but exhaustion can occur later, especially if the drug is injected. Sedatives may be taken in order to sleep. Ecstasy is an amphetamine drug, frequently taken for its stimulant effect by people at all-night clubs and parties. Deaths caused by cardiac arrhythmias and seizures have been reported.

Hallucinogens

Hallucinogens are taken for their mind-altering effects. Some are more dangerous than others.

Cannabis is obtained in dried leaf form, as resin, or a concentrated oil. It is usually smoked but can be ingested with food. It can cause a mild euphoria and sense of well-being. It is not addictive but association with the illegal drug culture can encourage the move to more harmful substances. Some dealers have been known to mix crack with cannabis in order to create addiction.

Lysergic acid diethylamide (LSD) causes hallucinating effects which last for for up to 12 hours. During that time the user may have a sense of disassociation from the body and be at risk from dangerous behaviour like trying to fly. LSD tablets are relatively cheap and readily available.

Solvents

The fumes from any volatile substance such as glue, antifreeze, lighter fuel, nail varnish remover, or aerosol propellants, can be inhaled from a plastic bag. The effects produced can look similar to intoxication with alcohol, but redness around the mouth, and running eyes and nose can be a give-away. There may be a history of poor school performance and truancy. Respiratory and renal failure can be caused by solvent abuse, as well as accidents due to dangerous behaviour or death from asphyxia or inhaled vomit.

Substance abuse is a major health problem. Practice nurses can provide information about addictive substances to parents and young people in the practice. A nurse may detect signs of possible solvent abuse, or note needle marks when taking a blood pressure or treating a wound. Patients may attend the surgery with physical complaints of weight loss, fatigue, gastric problems, blackouts, or accidents. There may also be reports of relationship problems, altered behaviour, absenteeism, financial problems, or self-neglect. Family members of people who misuse substances may be seen with frequent minor ailments which mask the true cause of their distress.

Eating disorders

Hunger is a physiological drive to eat in response to the body's needs for energy and nutrients. The appetite for certain foods can be indulged, or over-ridden, irrespective of the feelings of hunger. Social and familial customs and beliefs associated with food can affect an individual person's eating behaviour.

Anorexia nervosa

Sufferers from anorexia nervosa have a distorted body image which makes them strive for an abnormally low weight because they mistakenly believe that they are fat. Calorie intakes are strictly regulated and eating may be followed by induced vomiting. Female sufferers usually develop amenorrhoea as a result of starvation. Death can result if the process is not reversed.

Bulimia nervosa

With bulimia, periods of binge-eating are interspersed with vomiting, purging and violent exercise in an attempt to prevent weight gain. The shame and guilt associated with this loss of control reinforces the individual's poor self-image.

Practice nurses weigh patients during screening and well-person checks. Patients with anorexia nervosa may be identified by finding a very low BMI, but they are likely to deny having a problem. Patients with bulimia may have a normal weight/height ratio yet complain of being overweight. They may also have a past history of anorexia nervosa. The knuckles of patients with an eating disorder may be scarred by their teeth from persistently inducing vomiting. Referral is needed for specialised help for eating disorders.

Self-awareness in the caring professions

In order to provide empathetic support and care for patients and their families, nurses and doctors have to be able to deal with their own problems as human beings. Many people in the caring professions seem to have a particular need to be admired and respected; emotional conflict can arise if patients appear demanding or ungrateful. The stress experienced by some doctors may be reflected in their higher than average suicide rate[24].

All the members of the primary health care team should be encouraged to explore their own feelings and motivations. Clinical supervision and the review of critical incidents provide opportunities to discuss any matters of concern. The need for relaxation and stress-relieving activities applies as much to the professionals as to the patients. Co-counselling is a method whereby practitioners work in pairs to counsel each other. This is probably better done with a co-counsellor unconnected with the same GP practice. Other forms of counselling should be sought if they are needed.

Suggestions for reflection on practice

- How confident do you feel about looking after patients with mental health problems?
- Could the service they receive be improved?
- What system do you have for communicating with the community mental health team?

Further reading

Forster, S. (ed.) (2001) *The Role of the Mental Health Nurse*. Nelson Thornes, Cheltenham.

Royal College of Nursing (2001) *Managing Your Stress: A guide for nurses*. Royal College of Nursing, London.

Royal College of Nursing and NHS Executive (1998) *Safer Working in the Community*. Royal College of Nursing, London.

Thompson, T. & Mathias, P. (eds) (2000) *Lyttle's Mental Health and Disorder*. Bailliere Tindall, London.

UKCC (2000) *The Nursing, Midwifery and Health Visiting Contribution to the Continuing Care of People with Mental Health Problems. A review and UKCC action plan*. UKCC, London.

References

1. Martin, J.O. (1993) 'Holism' in the discourse of nursing. *Journal of Advanced Nursing*, **18**, 1688–95.
2. Atkin, K., Lunt, N., Parker, G. & Hirst, M. (1993) *Nurses Count: A National Survey of Practice Nurses*. SPRU, University of York.
3. Department of Health (1999) *National Service Framework for Mental Health–Modern Standards and Service Models*. HMSO, London.
4. Robb, B. (1967) *Sans Everything, A Case to Answer*. Nelson, London.
5. Secretary of State for Social Services (1978) *Report of the Committee of Enquiry into Normansfield Hospital*. HMSO, London.
6. Mind Fact Sheet. *The Care Programme Approach, www.mind.org.uk/information* (accessed 18/8/01).
7. Department of Health (1998) *Modernising Mental Health Services: safe, sound and supportive*. Department of Health, London.
8. Department of Health (2000) *The NHS Plan. A plan for investment. A plan for reform*. Department of Health, London.
9. Department of Health (2000) *Effective care coordination in mental health services*. Modernising the care programme approach – A policy booklet. HMSO, London.
10. Took, M. (2001) *Physical Care Needs of People with a Severe Mental Illness*. National Schizophrenia Fellowship Policy Statement No. 36.
11. Department of Health (1999) *Saving Lives: Our Healthier Nation*. DoH, London.
12. Department of Health (2000) *Reforming the Mental Health Act*. HMSO, London.
13. Walsh, M. & Kent, A. (2001) Violence and aggression. In: *Accident and Emergency Nursing* (4th edn.), pp. 184–9.
14. Gorman, J. (1997) *Understanding Post-Traumatic Stress Disorder*. MIND Publications.
15. Centre for Evidence-Based Mental Health (1999) *Depression guideline*, Appendix 1. *www.psychiatry.ox.ac.uk/cebmh/guidelines/depression* (accessed 17/8/01).
16. Whooley, M., Avins, A., Miranda, J. & Browner, W. (1997) Case-finding instruments for depression. Two questions are as good as many. *Journal of General Internal Medicine*, **12**, 439–45.
17. Geddes, J., Butler, R. & Warner, J. (2000) Recognizing and Treating Depression: The Latest Evidence, *Clinical Evidence*, **3**, 434–47.
18. Health Canada (2000) *Risk of Important Drug Interactions between St John's Wort and Prescription Drugs, www.hc-sc.gc.ca* (accessed 17/8/01).
19. Royal College of Nursing Scotland (1999) *Post Natal Depression*. Royal College of Nursing, Scotland.
20. Craddock, N. & Jones, I. (2001) Molecular genetics of bipolar disorder. *British Journal of Psychiatry*, 41 Suppl., S128–33.
21. De Hert, M. McKenzie, K. & Peuskens, J. (2001) Risk factors for suicide in young people sufferering from schizophrenia: a long-term follow-up study. *Schizophrenia Research*, **47** (2–3), 127–134.
22. Knight, R. (2001) *Creutzfeldt-Jakob disease*. NetDoctor factsheet. *www.netdoctor.co.uk/diseases/facts/cid*
23. Bandolier (2001) Consumption of different types of alcohol and mortality. *www.jr2.ox.ac.uk/bandolier/booth/hliving/Alctype* (accessed 9/10/01).
24. Lindemann, S., Laara, E., Hakko, H. & Lonnguist, J. (1996) A systematic review of gender-specific mortality in medical doctors. *British Journal of Psychiatry*, **169**, 274–9.

Useful address and web site

Mind (Mental health charity)
Registered Office
15–19 Broadway
London
E15 4BQ
Web site: *www.mind.org.uk*
(has links to all local branches and to other mental health charities and support associations)

Chapter 16
Supporting Patients with Chronic Diseases

The 1990 GP contract gave an impetus to the involvement of practice nurses in chronic disease management and nurses have demonstrated their ability in this field. Asthma, diabetes and hypertension were the first conditions with which large numbers of practice nurses developed expertise; followed by chronic obstructive pulmonary disease (COPD) and coronary heart disease (CHD). Epilepsy, skin diseases, gastointestinal conditions and blood disorders are ripe for more nurse involvement. No single nurse can expect to be sufficiently knowledgeable in all these subjects; yet the possibilities should not be over-looked. Many practices now employ more than one nurse, so there is nothing to stop each of them from specialising in different fields.

Any patient who attends a clinic at a GP surgery or health centre has a right to expect a uniformly high standard of service. The following points should be considered when writing the protocol or guidelines.

Aims for each clinic should be clear. Most clinics for chronic diseases will have similar aims:

- To help the patients and their families to understand the disease and take responsibility for its control
- To minimise the number of critical incidents
- To help the patients to lead as normal a life as possible.

Target groups may be all the patients who are known or suspected of having a particular disease, for example, all patients with asthma; or a subgroup, such as patients with type 2 diabetes.

Organisation – the way a clinic is to be organised. This will include:

- The amount of time to be allocated to each consultation
- The equipment, teaching aids and resources needed
- The record system to be used
- Education (in order to comply with the UKCC Code of Professional Conduct

and to ensure that a patient receives the best possible standard of service, a nurse must have acquired the appropriate knowledge and skills before attempting to run a clinic)

- A disease register and call/recall system is needed for each clinic
- Clerical support is necessary for contacting the patients and making appointments, so the nurse's time is used most effectively
- Outcome (how the achievements of the clinic will be audited).

Although the word *clinic* is used for convenience throughout this chapter, patients do not necessarily need to be seen at special clinic times; they may be seen during normal surgery hours. However, some sessions may be more convenient for the patients if arranged when other health professionals, such as a dietitian and chiropodist, are working in the practice. In some instances, depending on the degree of autonomy of the nurse, it may be preferable to have a doctor available during nurse-run clinics in case a medical examination, prescription, or hospital referral is needed.

Protocols for nurse-run clinics

A protocol can be tailored to minimum, moderate or maximum nursing input, in accordance with the practice nurse's knowledge and experience. Each protocol should specify the procedure to be followed at first and subsequent clinic appointments (see Chapter 3 for discussion on protocols, guidelines and clinical pathways).

Asthma

Asthma is an inflammatory disease of the airways characterised by narrowing of the bronchioles from:

- Inflammation and swelling of the mucosa
- Dysfunction of the smooth muscle in the walls of the bronchioles
- Thick mucus secretion.

The condition is intermittent and reversible; either spontaneously, or when the correct treatment is given.

Incidence

The incidence of asthma has been rising over the past decades, although the reasons are not fully understood. One in thirteen adults and one in eight children are currently estimated to be receiving treatment for asthma in the UK[1]. Therefore, in a practice with 8000 patients, up to 700 of them could be expected to have asthma. Children have the highest incidence of asthma but the condition can begin at any age. Three quarters of children with asthma may grow out of it, but unfortunately about 50% of those who do grow out of it can expect to develop asthma again in later life.

Causes

The trigger factors which precipitate asthma can be allergic or non-allergic. Anyone could have an asthma attack if exposed to a large enough trigger factor. People with asthma differ in having hyper-reactive airways, which react to even small contact with triggers. Allergic triggers include: house dust mites, pollen, moulds and spores, animal dander and chemicals. Non-allergic triggers can be: exercise, upper respiratory tract infections, cold air, cigarette smoke and emotional stress. The common cold is a very common trigger factor.

The aim of treatment is to suppress the bronchial hyper-reactivity, and the key to good control lies in concordance with the treatment. A patient who feels fit and well may be reluctant to continue with preventive therapy unless its importance is fully appreciated.

Asthma treatments (refer to the British National Formulary)

The British Thoracic Society has issued guidelines on a step-wise approach to treatment, so that the maximum control of asthma symptoms is achieved by using the most appropriate drugs[2]. Revised guidelines, to be published in 2002, are likely to recommend a reduction in the starting dose of inhaled steroids, especially in children[3].

Bronchodilators

The commonly used drugs in this field are the beta$_2$ stimulants, salbutamol (Ventolin) and terbutaline (Bricanyl) which act mainly by relaxing bronchial smooth muscle; thus relieving bronchoconstriction. For this reason broncho-dilators are called *reliever* drugs. Salmeterol (Serevent) is a longer-acting bronchodilator, useful in some cases for night-time and exercise-induced asthma. It should not be used as a reliever drug. This type of drug has been named a *protector* and should be used in conjunction with other asthma ther-apy. Oral preparations of theophylline (Slo-Phyllin, Uniphyllin Continus) or aminophylline (Phyllocontin Continus) are bronchodilators which can be used to relieve nocturnal or early-morning asthma. The dose has to be carefully adjusted for each patient, and the same brand of modified release drugs should be ordered each time. Generic prescribing is not appropriate for these drugs[4]. Regular blood tests are needed to maintain therapeutic drug levels.

Corticosteroids

Patients who need to use a reliever drug more than once a day usually require inhaled steroids to deal with the inflammation of the bronchial mucosa, e.g.

beclomethasone dipropionate, budesonide or fluticasone. Patients may have confused ideas about steroids and be reluctant to use them long term. It is important to explain their action as preventers and to ensure that patients know how to use them. Fungal infections of the mouth and throat are possible side effects. Patients can be advised to rinse the mouth after using the steroid inhaler. Children under five years and patients on high-dose steroids should use a spacer device for steroid inhalations. Fluticasone propionate (Flixotide) is an inhaled steroid which is said to have less systemic absorption and thus has a less detrimental effect on children's growth[5]. A short course of oral steroids may be prescribed as treatment for acute asthma. Occasionally patients require daily doses of oral steroids to control chronic asthma symptoms. Patients on maintenance therapy should be given a steroid card to carry, and be warned not to stop the drugs suddenly.

Combination therapies

Some inhalers have a combination of a bronchodilator with an anti-inflammatory preparation. These do not always contain the dosage needed by individual patients and may result in over- or under-use of one or other of the components. However, where the dosage is appropriate, a combined inhaler may aid concordance with the therapy.

Leukotriene receptor antagonists

Montelukast and zafirlukast are the newest additions to the range of asthma treatments. Their place in the management of asthma is still being evaluated. At present they may be used as additional treatments for mild to moderate asthma.

Inhaler devices

These include the following:

- Pressurised metered dose inhalers (with or without spacer devices)
- Breath actuated inhalers
- Dry powder devices.

Inhalers containing CFCs are being phased out in order to prevent further damage to the ozone layer[6]. Nurses should be familiar with the way all inhaler devices work. The NRTC sells a helpful video recording, *Devices in Detail*, which explains each system and how to teach patients to use them. Sales representatives will supply placebo inhalers for teaching purposes. Pressurised metered dose inhalers via a spacer, with a face mask if necessary, are recommended by the National Institute for Clinical Excellence (NICE) for the routine treatment of children under five years with chronic asthma[7].

Asthma clinic

Nurse education

The National Respiratory Training Centre (NRTC) at Warwick organises training for practice nurses. The name and scope of the organisation has changed over the years. It began in 1986, in a small house in Stratford-upon-Avon, as the National Asthma Training Centre, later expanded into the National Asthma and Respiratory Training Centre, with larger premises in Warwick, and then logically adopted the new name in September 2001. The centre now provides education in the management of respiratory diseases for nurses and doctors from around the world.

   The NRTC awards the Diploma in Asthma Care. A distance learning package is followed by consolidation and the examination at a regional training centre. Introductory and updating sessions are also run locally by the NRTC asthma trainers. The Diploma in Asthma Care attracts 24 CATS points at level 2. The ENB N83 asthma course leads to 20 credits at diploma level.

The equipment needed

This includes:

- Scales and height chart
- PEFR meter and mouthpiece for adults and children
- PEFR prediction calculator or charts
- Bronchodilator for reversibility tests
- Placebo inhalers for teaching inhaler techniques
- Explanatory booklets for adults and children
- Instruction leaflets, diagrams and peak flow diaries
- Information about voluntary organisations and other services.

The practice computer may have an asthma clinic template. Many of the asthma drug companies provide useful materials for nurses and patients. Primary care organisations usually have guidelines for working with the pharmaceutical industry to ensure that no undue pressure is applied to promote particular products. The National Asthma Campaign funds asthma research, supplies literature and runs the Asthma Helpline telephone service. Information about asthma can also be obtained via the Internet. The NRTC sells a range of literature and teaching aids.

Protocol

The NRTC has produced guidelines for minimum, medium and maximum nurse involvement as part of the distance learning package. The protocol should specify how much of the following procedures will be undertaken by the nurse.

Procedure for a first consultation

For a patient with suspected, or newly diagnosed asthma use the following guidelines.

History   This will include:

- Past medical history: including allergies or eczema
- Asthma history: age at onset, trigger factors, symptoms and treatments used
- Family history: including atopic conditions
- Social history: smoking and exercise, occupation and any relationship of the asthma to work
- Current medication: are inhalers used?

Tests and examination   This will include:

- General health assessment: to identify any risk factors and establish a baseline (include BP, height, weight and urinalysis). Steroids can affect growth in children and precipitate diabetes in some patients.
- Peak expiratory flow rate (see Chapter 6). Compare with the predicted PEFR.

Diagnostic tests (if asthma is not yet confirmed)   The following may be used:

- Reversibility test: record the PEFR immediately before and ten minutes after inhaling salbutamol or terbutaline. If the PEFR improves by 5% or more this is diagnostic of asthma.
- Exercise tolerance test (if appropriate for the patient): record the PEFR before and after six minute's exercise. PEFR should be recorded at five minute intervals for 15 minutes. The diagnosis of asthma will be confirmed if the peak flow falls by 15% or more. Recovery may be spontaneous but if necessary an inhaled bronchodilator can be used.
- Serial peak flow readings: ask the patient to keep a diary of twice daily readings and a record of any symptoms. A 5% difference between the morning and evening reading is normal, but differences of 15% or more indicate asthma.
- Steroid trial: to see if a significant improvement is achieved, when reversibility tests have been unimpressive.

General health promotion (see Chapter 9)   This will include:

- Discuss the factors which may affect the asthma most.
- Explain the nature of asthma so that the patient can comprehend. Parents of children with asthma can have their lives severely disrupted. They need a chance to talk about their anxieties and to learn as much as possible about asthma. Asthma storybooks can be used for small children.
- Explain how the treatment works and how and when to use it.

- Identify the trigger factors to be avoided, e.g. smoking by parents.
- Ensure that patients and parents understand the signs of worsening asthma and know what to do.
- Provide information about the voluntary societies.
- Offer immunisation against pneumococcal pneumonia and influenza.
- Inhaler technique: select the most suitable device and teach the parent or patient how to use it.

PEFR monitoring   Teach the patient how to monitor and record his/her peak flow at home (if able to use a peak flow meter).

Procedure for subsequent visits

Monitor progress   Use the following guidelines:

- Discuss the asthma diary and any significant entries
- Discuss other lifestyle factors, e.g. smoking
- Enquire about any work or schooling missed
- Discuss any problems with the medication.

Observations   Observe the following:

- Check the PEFR and compare with the predicted rate
- Check the patient's inhaler technique, re-teach if necessary, or consider an alternative delivery system
- Give praise generously when it is due.

Education   This will include the following:

- Ask the patient or parent to explain what he/she understands about asthma and its treatment. Gently correct any misunderstandings. It is important to be sure that the patient really has understood. What seems very basic physiology to a nurse, may be quite incomprehensible to a lay-person.
- Patients who are familiar with their asthma can be given self-management cards which tell them what to do in particular circumstances. For example: if PEFR is below 70% then repeat relief treatment and double the dose of inhaled steroid; if PEFR is below 50% then start course of oral steroids and call the GP or asthma clinic nurse.

Records   Keep records as follows:

- Patients who are able to do so should keep their own asthma diaries of peak flow and symptoms

- The National Asthma Campaign produces treatment cards for patients to carry, and for children to take to school
- Computer records can make audit easier.

The nurse's records must be kept in accordance with the UKCC guidelines for *Standards of Records and Record Keeping* (see Chapter 2).

Audit   This may be done as follows:

- Statistics can be collated about the number of patients on the asthma register, the percentage who attended a clinic in the past year and how many are receiving prophylactic therapy
- The number and cost of repeat prescriptions for inhalers can be monitored: if requests are too frequent, or infrequent, the inhalers may not be being used correctly
- Emergency hospital admissions or treatments for asthma can be analysed to see if they could have been prevented by better asthma management.

Anonymous questionnaires can help in discovering how many patients have asthma symptoms, and how well they use the treatment. Patient satisfaction questionnaires will show whether services for patients with asthma need to be improved.

Chronic obstructive pulmonary disease (COPD)

About 26 000 people died from COPD in 1992, as opposed to the 1700 who died from asthma[8]. Yet it is only in recent years that COPD has begun to receive the same sort of attention as asthma. This could be because asthma often affects younger people and usually responds well to therapy, and/or because COPD is closely linked with smoking, so the disease was considered to be self-inflicted, and also because treatment outcomes were less certain. Whatever the reasons, COPD has been receiving greater attention since the mid-1990s.

The National Asthma Training Centre was renamed the National Asthma and Respiratory Training Centre, when the organisation expanded to cover other respiratory conditions, and started running a distance learning course on COPD. The British Thoracic Society published *COPD Guidelines* in 1997 and the disease was given a higher priority in primary care[9]. The NHS Plan in the year 2000 expressed the intention to step up smoking cessation services and primary care organisations made help for smokers a priority in health improvement programmes around the country. *Chronic Obstructive Pulmonary Disease in Primary Care*, a manual produced by the NARTC and endorsed by the GPs In Asthma Group (GPIAG) is a useful resource for general practice[10].

COPD is the term used for airflow obstruction caused by chronic bronchitis and emphysema. It is a slowly progressive disorder of respiration, which usually develops in later life. Smoking is the single most important cause, although not all smokers develop COPD. The symptoms of breathlessness, cough and increased sputum gradually affect the ability to perform the normal activities of daily living. The possibility of lung cancer should not be ruled out in patients with worsening symptoms. Small airways disease or chronic asthma can also result in COPD.

- *Chronic bronchitis* is characterised by excessive mucus production – the 'smoker's cough'. Acute exacerbations with infected sputum requiring antibiotics, are more common in the winter months, although not all exacerbations are caused by infection; there may be an increased airflow obstruction causing dyspnoea and wheeze.
- *Emphysema* The airspaces at the end of the terminal bronchioles become enlarged and their walls are destroyed, leaving less surface area for the exchange of gases.

Clinical signs may not be obvious in the earlier stages of COPD but as the disease progresses the oxygenation of the blood can be affected. Compensation in the form of an increased red cell count causes increased viscosity of the blood, which carries the added risk of deep vein thrombosis and pulmonary embolism. Severe hypoxia causes cyanosis and mental confusion. Right heart failure develops as a result of pulmonary hypertension in COPD. The pulmonary capillaries become constricted and oxygenation of the blood is impaired. The right ventricle becomes hypertrophied from trying to pump blood through the damaged lungs, and eventually fails, leading in turn, to an increased systemic venous pressure and peripheral oedema. Respiratory failure may occur eventually.

Care is needed with oxygen therapy because the respiratory centre can sometimes be depressed further by oxygen. Hypoxia can become the stimulus to respiration in some people with COPD; rather than the build up of carbon dioxide, which is the normal respiratory stimulus.

Treatment (see *British National Formulary*)

The aims of the early recognition and management of COPD are to:

- Alleviate the symptoms
- Prevent the more severe complications of the condition
- Improve the patient's quality of life
- Prevent premature death.

Smoking cessation (see Chapter 9)

Lung function reduces naturally with age and the rate of decline can be accelerated by smoking. The damage caused by smoking cannot be reversed but the rate of decline can be slowed significantly. Hence the enthusiasm for helping people to quit smoking.

Bronchodilators

Beta$_2$ agonists may give a significant improvement in symptoms, even if the patient has a very limited degree of reversibility. A bronchodilator trial over three to four weeks is recommended. There is some evidence that the combination of a beta$_2$ agonists with an anticholinergic is more effective than either given singly[11].

Corticosteroids

The value of steroids in COPD is under review. The BTS guidelines for COPD recommend steroid trials for patients with moderate or severe COPD.

Pulmonary rehabilitation

Some patients with COPD may be helped by a rehabilitation programme. Physiotherapists can teach appropriate exercises to maximise lung function and retain mobility; occupational therapists can help with adaptations to the home and advise about ways to manage the everyday activities. Local respiratory support groups may help patients to maintain the progress made through rehabilitation and reduce social isolation. A practice nurse needs to have information about the national and local services for patients with respiratory conditions.

The role of the practice nurse

The role of practice nurses in COPD will depend on the education and experience of each nurse. Where a practice owns a spirometer, the practice nurse should have training in how to use it. The NRTC trainers run spirometry essential skills workshops. Many patients with COPD may be wrongly diagnosed as having asthma. For this reason it might be better to run a combined respiratory clinic in general practice, although the diseases are separated in this chapter for convenience.

COPD clinic

Organisation

Organisation needs to include:

- Disease register of patients with COPD
- Call and recall system for appointments

- Recall system for influenza immunisation
- Spirometer
- Materials for teaching, placebo inhalers
- Appropriate record system.

Clinic procedure

Clinic procedure will include:

- General health and respiratory history
- Smoking cessation advice and support (see Chapter 9, Health Promotion)
- Spirometry
- Bronchodilator reversibility testing
- Possible steroid trial
- Treatment as appropriate
- Pneumococcal immunisation
- Referral as appropriate.

Outcomes

Outcomes may include:

- Percentage of patients on the register who attended a COPD clinic in a year
- Improvements in lung function and/or quality of life in patients with COPD
- Number of patients who successfully stopped smoking
- Patient satisfaction with the service
- Number of emergency admissions with COPD.

Some of the data may be statistical, while other information, such as patient satisfaction or sense of well-being, will be more subjective. Both types of information can be used to demonstrate the value of a clinic. A reduction in the number of emergency admissions could demonstrate that the management of COPD is being effective.

Diabetes mellitus

A practice with 8000 patients can expect to have about 160 known diabetic patients, but there may be almost as many again who are undiagnosed. Hence the need for screening. The UK national average is between 2–3% of the population. Diabetes is a chronic metabolic condition caused by a deficiency of insulin, or resistance to its effect classified as:

- Type 1 diabetes mellitus (previously called insulin-dependent diabetes). This is due to the destruction of beta cells in the pancreatic islets of Langerhans resulting in the loss of insulin production. Children and adults under the age of 40 years are most commonly affected. The treatment is by regular injections of insulin. The aim is to maintain blood glucose levels as near to normal as possible.

- Type 2 diabetes (previously called non-insulin dependent diabetes or maturity onset diabetes), results from either diminished insulin secretion or an increased peripheral resistance to the action of insulin. The cause is still uncertain. It usually occurs in later life and is often associated with obesity or a family history of diabetes. Patients of Asian or Afro-Caribbean origin are more susceptible to develop this condition. Women with a history of gestational diabetes are also in the risk group. The treatment may be by diet and exercise alone, or diet, exercise and hypoglycaemic drugs. Type 2 diabetes is not a mild form of the disease; the complications can be just as serious as those of type 1 diabetes and good metabolic control is equally important.

Diagnosis

A practice nurse might be the first person to discover that a patient has diabetes; either during routine screening or because the patient has particular risk factors or symptoms. All pregnant women must be screened. Anyone complaining of thirst, polyuria or nocturia; who has recurrent boils or fungal infections, tiredness, paraesthesia, visual changes or ischaemic problems should be tested. A random blood glucose >11.1 mmol/l or a fasting glucose > 7 mmol/l is indicative of diabetes[12]. The patient will need to be referred to the GP, and the education process should be started. In some cases a glucose tolerance test may be needed to confirm the diagnosis (see Chapter 6, Diagnostic tests and investigations).

Patients with type 1 diabetes are usually referred to a diabetologist but the practice/PCT policy should determine which groups of patients are referred. Shared care between the hospital and the practice diabetic clinic can be a good way to make the best use of valuable resources and provide a consistently high level of service.

Initial patient education

Most patients will be shocked by the diagnosis of diabetes and will not retain very much information initially. A straightforward explanation about the condition can be backed up by written information to be read at home. The patient should be given verbal and written information on healthy eating, and an appointment to see the dietitian. Special diet foods are not necessary. Healthy food for someone with diabetes is the same as healthy food for everyone else. The practice dietitian will usually provide a sample diet sheet to photocopy for patients, covering the following points:

- Eat regular meals containing starchy foods, e.g. potatoes, bread, cereals (foods high in fibre take longer to digest, so do not increase the blood sugar as much as rapidly digested refined carbohydrates).
- Have less sugary foods or drinks. Use sugar-reduced products instead.
- Eat only small amounts of fried or fatty foods. Use reduced fat products and skimmed or semi-skimmed milk.
- Eat at least five portions of fruit and vegetables a day.
- Use only a small amount of salt (to help avoid high blood pressure).
- Drink alcohol in moderation and avoid drinking on an empty stomach (alcohol can lower the blood glucose level)[13].

Before the diagnosis of diabetes was made, patients with polydipsia may have been compounding the problem by drinking large amounts of lemonade or sweetened fruit juice and squashes, in an attempt to quench their thirst. A high blood glucose can also affect the lens of the eye resulting in blurred vision. Patients should be advised not to buy new glasses until the diabetes has been controlled and reasonable glycaemic levels attained.

The patient should be offered another appointment as soon as possible after diagnosis for education about the nature of the condition and how to manage it. This should include:

- Reinforcement of the information about the nature of diabetes and how good glycaemic control can reduce the risk of complications
- Advice about healthy living (smoking, alcohol and exercise)
- The need to attain or maintain a normal body weight
- How to monitor and record blood glucose levels (diabetes is a life-long condition, which the patient needs to understand and take control of)
- The importance of a regular health check and an annual medical review
- The importance of foot care
- Information about Diabetes UK, previously the British Diabetic Association (membership gives patients access to a lot of helpful information and support).

Diabetes UK also has a professional membership section, which anyone running a diabetic clinic would find useful.

Treatment

Diet

See above for general advice. A dietitian will make a full dietary assessment for each patient and advise accordingly.

Oral hypoglycaemic agents

Oral hypoglycaemic preparations may be prescribed once it has been shown that diet and exercise alone does not control the blood sugar level.

Sulphonylurea drugs Drugs such as glibenclamide, gliclazide, glipizide and tolbutamide act by stimulating the remaining insulin secreting cells to perform more efficiently. All these drugs can cause weight gain, and are therefore not the first choice for clinically obese patients. Sulphonylureas can cause gastro-intestinal disturbances, and also on rare occasions hypoglycaemia or blood disorders.

Biguanides Metformin acts by increasing the peripheral uptake of glucose. It can be added to the sulphonylurea treatment, or used instead of it. It may also be prescribed in combination with one of the newer drugs.

Thiazolidiniones Rosiglitazone and Pioglitazone are more recently introduced drugs, which act by reducing the peripheral resistance to insulin. They have both been subject to appraisal by the National Institute for Clinical Excellence (NICE) and the guidelines recommend that they may be used in combination with metformin (preferably), or a sulphonylurea drug, as an alternative to insulin for patients who cannot take a combination of metformin and a sulphonylurea and whose blood glucose is not controlled[14-15]. The liver function of patients taking thiazolidione drugs should be monitored because they can be hepatotoxic.

Other antidiabetic drugs Acarbose and guar gum may both be used to delay carbohydrate absorption.

Insulin This has to be administered parenterally because, being a protein, it would be digested if given orally. There are many different types of insulin, classified either according to their speed of action, or their source:

* Short- medium- and long-acting insulins can be obtained individually or in various combinations
* Insulins derived from pork or beef pancreas, or synthetically produced human insulins.

A patient's religious beliefs must be taken into account when prescribing insulin. Jewish and Muslim people cannot use porcine insulin, and Hindus are forbidden to use insulin derived from beef.

   Good glucose control has been said to reduce the risk of complications, but the tighter the control, the greater the risk of hypoglycaemia[16]. Patients and the people close to them need to recognise the signs and symptoms of hypo-glycaemia and know what action to take if it occurs.

Diabetic clinics

Practice nurse education

Nurses who run diabetic clinics should have adequate training, for example, the ENB 928 Short Course in Diabetes, as a minimum, or ENB N97 Diabetes

Nursing in the Primary Health Care Setting or equivalent, as an ideal. The Diabetes Training Centre distance learning package provides a sound grounding and qualification at diploma level. Diabetes nurse specialists often run updating sessions for practice nurses, and will advise on setting up nurse-led diabetic clinics.

Resources

Diabetes UK has published updated guidelines for the management of diabetes in primary care. These may be updated again after the National Service Framework for Diabetes has been published. Blood glucose monitoring is an important aspect of diabetes care. Therefore it is essential that all healthcare professionals engaged in blood glucose monitoring have been trained adequately and understand how to use specific blood glucose meters correctly. Blood glucose meters must be kept clean and calibrated with each batch of test strips. Appropriate quality control measures must be taken for each machine. Disposable finger pricking devices should be used in a practice setting, to prevent the transmission of blood-borne diseases.

Services

There should be arrangements for prompt access to a dietitian and chiropodist. Local social services or district nursing may be required for patients with any disabilities associated with diabetes. All patients require an ophthalmic examination at least annually, and patients with severe visual problems may need to be referred to the social services sensory impairment team. Anyone with impaired mobility may require an occupational therapy assessment. Diabetes UK has produced a booklet telling patients of their rights and responsibilities and what diabetes care to expect from the NHS[17]. Special holidays can be arranged to teach children how to lead a normal life with diabetes.

Procedure for initial consultations

A practice nurse will carry out the tests and investigations specified in the protocol. The initial assessment should cover the following areas:

History

Social history   Check the following:

- Home situation and family support available.
- Lifestyle factors, such as smoking, alcohol consumption, diet and exercise.

- Occupation and driving. Type 1 diabetes may preclude some occupations, such as driving heavy goods or public service vehicles. The licensing centre at Swansea must be notified about the diagnosis of diabetes, and the motor insurers should also be informed.

Medical history   Check the following:

- Previous illnesses and operations
- Family history: history of diabetes, ischaemic conditions, eye problems or hypertension
- Contraception – a higher dose combined pill may be required if oral hypo-glycaemic drugs are used.

Examination   Check the following:

- Weight, height and BMI: patients with type 1 diabetes may have lost weight. Patients with type 2 diabetes may be overweight.
- Urinalysis for:
  - glucose
  - protein
  - ketones
  - infection.
- Blood pressure – because hypertension increases the risks for CHD and stroke. Hypertension may also be a sign of nephropathy. A postural drop may signify autonomic neuropathy.
- Feet: check the skin condition and circulation, and need for chiropody. Peripheral neuropathy and micro-vascular damage can lead to gangrene if any traumatic lesions or ulcers are not detected early.
- Eyes: check visual acuity with spectacles, if worn.

Blood tests   Baseline: full blood count, urea and electrolytes, serum creatinine, plasma glucose, liver function tests, fasting lipid profile, thyroid function tests.

Education for patients

Discussions should take place to ensure all the staff in general practice and the diabetic unit give consistent information and advice. The amount of information to be given at each visit needs to be judged carefully. More frequent appointments may be required during the initial period of adjustment. Consider the following:

- The patient and family need to understand the reasons for maintaining good blood sugar control, how to monitor the blood sugar levels and to test the urine for ketones

- Advice and information are needed on dietary management and lifestyle adjustments, such as dinner parties or business lunches
- A patient stabilised on insulin needs help to master the self-administration of injections and advice on care of the skin
- Hypoglycaemia must be explained, so the patient knows how to recognise the symptoms and take appropriate action to raise the blood sugar level to normal limits
- Patients must know what to do if they are ill (a supply of *Sick Day Guideline* leaflets can be obtained from Diabetes UK), see Appendix 3
- Preconceptual counselling and close monitoring during pregnancy are essential
- Ways of coping with travel might need to be discussed (see Chapter 11)
- A patient whose job is affected may need to be referred for specialist employment advice
- Daily low-dose aspirin (75 mg) is recommended for patients aged over thirty with a blood pressure below 150/90 mm Hg to reduce the risk of cardio-vascular disease[18].

Procedure for a routine review

The following points need to be considered:

- Discuss the general health of the patient and any problems experienced.
- Weigh the patient and encourage positive progress towards a normal BMI.
- Test urine for glucose, protein and ketones. Send an MSU if any proteinuria is present.
- Screening for microalbuminuria may be carried out. Persistent micro-albuminuria is a predictor for diabetic nephropathy.
- Take a blood sample of glycosylated haemoglobin to check the long-term blood sugar control. (This may be before the consultation, so the result is available.)
- Review the results of home blood or urine testing.
- Measure and record blood pressure. Levels of 140/80 mmHg or below are the ideal for people with diabetes. Treatment should be considered for patients with levels consistently above this level. The blood pressure should also be measured when the patient is standing, to detect orthostatic hypotension.
- Discuss any problems with the medication or diet.
- Assess the patient's understanding of diabetes and its management. Correct any misunderstandings.
- Discuss any sexual problems. Erectile dysfunction commonly occurs with diabetes.
- Teach, as required, anything the patient is unsure about:
  - the diet, blood glucose monitoring, urinalysis, foot care, insulin injections, hypoglycaemia
  - coping with illness.

Annual review

In addition to the routine review procedure the annual review should provide:

- A full medical examination including the feet, injection sites, peripheral pulses and fundi.
- The diabetic control and treatment should be reviewed. (Blood tests for glucose, HbA$_1$, lipids and creatinine can be taken beforehand, so that the results are ready for the review.)
- Assessment for complications. An early morning urine specimen may be sent for albumin creatinine ratio (ACR) to test for diabetic nephropathy.
- Examination of the eyes. Patients should be advised that they will be unable to drive for several hours after the pupils have been dilated for fundoscopy. The drops should not be used for patients who have glaucoma or a history of eye surgery. If fundoscopy is not undertaken in the practice, the patient can be examined free of charge by an ophthalmic optician.

Records

The practice diabetes register must be kept up to date and the patients may also be entered in a district diabetes register. Patients should be encouraged to keep records of their home monitoring and treatment. Patient-held shared care cards allow good communication between the hospital service and the practice. An entry should be made in the patients' records at each consultation.

Defaulters need to be followed up and alternative arrangements suggested if the clinic times are unsuitable. The management of diabetes in teenagers can be challenging at times. Some teenagers need extra encouragement to take an active part in self-management. A chronic disease can lead to a degree of resistance at this age because the need for conformity with the peer group is so strong. Parents can feel torn between the need to protect their children and the need to allow them increasing independence, especially if the young people themselves are refusing to take a responsible attitude towards their disease. The natural anxiety for the welfare of their children can make some parents overprotective; thereby creating conflict in the home.

Assessing the success of the clinic

Statistics can be compiled about the patients with diabetes registered with the practice, and be compared with the predicted number for the practice size. Details of clinic attendance, waiting times and defaulters can be collated. Audit the percentage of patients with diabetes who have an annual review and the frequency that certain procedures were carried out: blood pressure measurement, foot checks, blood tests, and eye examinations. Other suggestions for audit include: the percentage of overweight patients who succeeded in losing weight, the levels of glycaemic control achieved, the percentage of patients with diabetes taking aspirin and the number of emergency admissions to hospital. A questionnaire and suggestions for improvements to the service can help to determine patient satisfaction.

Hypertension

High blood pressure increases the risk of heart disease and strokes and can cause particular problems for patients with diabetes. The pressure which the blood exerts on the artery walls is created in two main ways: by the cardiac output – the force of the blood expelled during systole, and the peripheral resistance – the calibre of the arterioles. The blood pressure is controlled centrally by the hypothalamus. Pressure receptors in the aorta and carotid arteries send stimuli to the vasomotor centre, which in turn controls the peripheral resistance via the autonomic nervous system. The cardiac centre controls the rate and contractility of the heart.

The kidneys, which require sufficient pressure for filtration, have their own system for raising the blood pressure if it is too low. Renin is secreted by cells near the glomeruli, which starts a chain reaction. As a result of which angiotensin II increases the peripheral resistance by vasoconstriction and stimulates the adrenal cortex to secrete aldosterone, which increases the blood volume through the retention of sodium and water in the renal tubules.

In 80% of patients with high blood pressure, no cause can be established. This is primary or essential hypertension. There may be an inherited tendency but lifestyle factors also play a part. Secondary hypertension results from another medical condition – neurological, cardiac, renal or endocrine. Hypertension can be life-threatening during pregnancy.

Diagnosis

Blood pressure increases naturally with age and in response to exercise or anxiety. The British Hypertension Society has made recommendations for the treatment of patients with a persistently raised blood pressure[19]. The criteria are stricter for treating patients with diabetes or cardiovascular disease. No patient should be diagnosed as hypertensive on one isolated reading. The reading should usually be repeated on three separate occasions, after resting for at least ten minutes each time. Home monitoring may be needed for patients with suspected 'white coat syndrome'[20].

Treatment

Mild hypertension might be managed by patients, without any CVS or end-target disease, by changes in lifestyle such as stopping smoking, increased exercise, reduced alcohol intake, healthy eating and weight loss if obese. Medical or surgical treatment may be possible for any condition causing secondary hypertension. Drug therapy is usually required to control more severe hypertension. The drug treatments include:

- Thiazide diuretics: e.g. bendrofluazide 2.5 mg may be used alone to control mild hypertension, or be used in conjunction with other drugs.
- Beta-blockers: e.g. atenolol or propranolol lowers blood pressure by reducing the cardiac activity and/or the peripheral resistance, depending on the selectivity of the drug used.
- Calcium channel blockers: e.g. nifedipine or diltiazem prevent the influx of calcium ions across the membrane of smooth muscle, and so reduces vaso-constriction. Some also affect the cardiac output by decreasing the myo-cardial contractility.
- Angiotensin-converting enzyme (ACE) inhibiters: e.g. captopril, enalapril or lisinopril prevent the conversion of angiotensin I to angiotensin II in response to renin secretion; thus preventing peripheral vasoconstriction and aldosterone secretion.

More powerful drugs, hydralazine or prazosin, may be used for patients with severe hypertension which is not controlled by other means.

Hypertension clinics

Nurse education

Training may be obtained through local study days or practice nurse courses. Diploma level courses or distance learning packages on coronary heart disease include all aspects of hypertension management. Completion of such a course should equip the nurse with the necessary knowledge and skills to provide a high quality service to patients, as well as providing evidence of the standard of learning achieved.

Equipment

Mercury sphygmomanometers are likely to be phased out by the year 2005 because of the toxic effects of mercury. Replacement machines should meet and be maintained to the approved standards[21]. The following points should be considered while mercury sphygmomanometers are still being used:

- Cuffs must be available in child's, normal adult and large adult sizes. A thigh cuff is not suitable for an arm.
- The rubber tubing and balloon should not be perished and the valve must be able to control the release of air at 2 mm a second.
- The sphygmomanometer must be cleaned and maintained regularly.
- Access to a mercury spillage kit is required in case of accidents (see Chapter 4).

The hypertension protocol should be drawn up according to the knowledge and experience of the nurse.

Procedure for a first visit

The following procedure should be used:

History   Note the following information:

- Social history: including smoking, alcohol, diet, salt consumption, exercise, occupation and stress factors.
- Medical history: including asthma, diabetes, allergies, heart or kidney disease.
- Family history: including hypertension, CVS disease, diabetes and renal disease.

Investigations   Make the following investigations:

- Blood pressure recordings. The patient should be seated and have rested for ten minutes. There should be no restrictive clothing around the arm.
- Height, weight and BMI. Dietary advice is needed if the patient is over-weight.
- Urinalysis: for glycosuria and protein.
- Blood tests:
    - Serum creatinine, urea and electrolytes for renal function
    - Fasting lipids to detect hyperlidaemia which increases risks for CHD and stroke
    - Fasting glucose if diabetes is a possibility.
- Electrocardiogram to show any evidence of left ventricular hypertrophy.

Action   The following action may be required:

- According to the BP, investigation results and protocol.
- Arrange recall date.

Patient education   The education of any patient with a medical condition requires good interpersonal skills. With hypertension in particular, dire warnings about strokes and heart attacks are more likely to be counter-productive. Anxiety about the reading can cause a significant rise in blood pressure; even a look of concentration on a nurse's face may alarm a patient. Patients with access to the Internet may seek out their own information and wish to discuss it, but all patients will require suitable explanations and liter-ature to back up any information given.

Procedure for subsequent visits

Check information   Enquire about:

- Any changes in the patient's general health, lifestyle or social situation since the last visit
- Any side effects from the medication (if used), i.e. nausea, diarrhoea, giddiness, lassitude, faintness, erectile dysfunction, cold extremities
- Has the patient been taking the drugs (if prescribed)?

Investigations   These will include:

- Blood pressure – take two readings and calculate the mean pressure
- Check the patient's weight and calculate the BMI
- Check the pulse rate (if beta-blockers used).

The nurse must know the blood pressure levels at which he/she is expected to refer the patient back to the doctor.

Education   Include the following:

- Check the patient's understanding of hypertension and any treatment prescribed. Correct any misunderstandings and make sure that the patient is aware of the need to report any side effects, and not to stop the medication suddenly.
- Encourage the continuation of appropriate lifestyle changes.

Records

Computer records are most commonly used. A patient-held card is useful if a patient is also being treated at a hospital. It can be infuriating when a patient with well-controlled hypertension has his/her treatment discontinued in hospital because the blood pressure is found to be normal.

Recall

The frequency of appointments will depend on the degree of hypertension and its control. The recall system should be able to identify defaulters, so they do not slip through the net. All adults aged under 80 years should have blood pressure measured at least once every five years and annual checks are recommended for those with any history of blood pressure outside the normal range.

Audit

In addition to the clinic statistics an audit may cover:

- The amount by which patients' blood pressures are reduced. The BHS audit standards for BP levels in the surgery are < 150/90 in non-diabetic patients and < 140/85 in patients with diabetes. Targets for both systolic and diastolic readings should be reached[22].
- The incidence of heart attack and stroke in hypertensive patients, with a comparison between those who did, or did not, attend the hypertension clinic.
- The incidence of side effects with antihypertensive drugs.

Coronary heart disease (CHD)

The *National Service Framework for Coronary Heart Disease* sets out twelve standards for the prevention, diagnosis and treatment of CHD[23]. Some of these standards apply to society in general and others to hospital and the emergency services. However, practice nurses should be aware of the specific standards that involve primary care. These include:

- Reducing heart disease in the population by reducing risk factors and inequalities, and by increasing the number of ex-smokers
- Identifying people with established cardiovascular disease and offering secondary prevention measures
- Primary prevention of CHD by targeting people at risk and offering appropriate advice and treatment
- Aspirin to be given to people thought to be having a heart attack and thrombolysis within one hour of calling for professional help
- People with symptoms of angina to receive appropriate investigations and treatment
- Patients with suspected heart failure to receive appropriate investigations and treatment
- Patients admitted with CHD to be offered cardiac rehabilitation and secondary prevention to reduce the risk of further cardiac problems and to help them return to a normal life.

Practices are required to maintain a working CHD disease register and to work to a locally agreed protocol for the assessment, treatment and follow-up of patients with cardiovascular disease. Annual audit data is required to demonstrate the achievement of the goals of the NSF.

CHD is yet another field in which practice nurses are proving their ability. CHD nurses have been employed by many primary care organisations to help general practices comply with the standards of the NSF. Many of these nurses organise teaching sessions for the practices and will provide support to practice nurses in setting up CHD/heart failure clinics within their own surgeries. Cardiac nurses may also help to run such clinics.

Primary healthcare team members can also undertake distance learning courses. The DTC Primary Care Training Centre runs a CHD programme accredited by Huddersfield University, which can be satellited if enough people wish to take the course within a locality. The British Heart Foundation Heartsave programme is another distance learning package which gives an excellent education in all aspects of CHD.

Coronary heart disease clinic

All patients should have an annual review. This can be done in the practice by an appropriately trained practice nurse or cardiac nurse; thus saving the patient from a trip to the hospital and helping to reduce hospital waiting times. The review should include:

- General health check – blood pressure, weight, height, BMI and ankle oedema
- Investigations – urinalysis for protein, ECG, blood tests: FBC, glucose, lipids, creatinine (urea and electolytes if taking diuretics or ACE inhibitors)
- Medication review – is the patient on adequate doses, are they being taken correctly, are there any side effects?
- Advice on lifestyle – smoking, physical activity, diet (salt and fat in particular), driving
- Advice on managing chest pain/shortness of breath
- Discussion of any concerns, e.g. employment.

How to manage chest pain/angina

As waiting lists for coronary intervention can be up to 18 months, there are many patients who have to live with angina until they are seen in secondary care. Emergency hospital admissions may be reduced by teaching people how to recognise the signs and symptoms of angina. Most patients will have glyceryl trinitrate in tablet or spray form. Patients with tablets need to know that they expire after eight weeks and need to be replaced by fresh ones. GTN can be purchased over the counter in most pharmacies without a prescription.

Information for patients on how to use GTN   Make sure that patients know how to:

- Prevent an attack:
  - If they know when an attack may occur (i.e. after exercise or exertion) one tablet can be placed under the tongue and allowed to dissolve, or one puff can be sprayed under the tongue, five to ten minutes before the event.

(Many patients become expert at knowing what precipitates angina, so they can be taught that preventing an attack is better than experiencing it.)

- Relieve an attack:
  - Stop what they are doing, sit down and try to relax. This may relieve some of the pain.

- If the pain continues, place one tablet under the tongue and allow it to dissolve or spray one puff under the tongue.
- Wait five to ten minutes and if the pain is not relieved, repeat the GTN tablet or spray.
- Seek medical help if they still feel chest pain 20 minutes after it started.

Heart failure

The diagnosis of heart failure in primary care can be difficult. All patients with suspected heart failure should have an ECG in the first instance but heart failure cannot be ruled out, even if the ECG is normal. A chest x-ray can show the heart size but will not confirm heart failure. The gold standard is the echocardiogram, but the waiting time for this procedure can be many months. So if heart failure is suspected, the patient should be started on the appropriate treatment and the response monitored. A good response to treatment is indicative of a correct diagnosis. Patients with heart failure account for 5% of all elderly care admissions and many are re-admitted within six months of discharge. Follow-up in the community can improve the patient's quality of life and help to prevent some admissions to hospital.

Heart failure clinic

All patients should be included in an actively used heart failure register. They should be reviewed every 6–12 months, depending on their condition.

Clinic procedure

This should be as follows:

- All medication should be reviewed at each consultation. (Referral to secondary care may be needed for the initiation of some therapies, e.g. beta-blockers.)
- Blood tests, according to the practice guidelines – FBC, urea and electrolytes.
- Teach patients to recognise the signs of increasing heart failure such as weight gain, ankle oedema, fatigue, increasing shortness of breath and to seek advice and medical assistance before they become acutely unwell. All patients with heart failure should weigh themselves three times a week, if stable, or daily if less stable. The GP or nurse should be contacted if a weight gain is more than 1–2 kg in 24 hours.
- Advise on physical activity or refer for specialist advice if required. All patients with heart failure should be encouraged to exercise.
- Advise on diet. Low salt intake will help reduce fluid retention. Smaller more frequent meals are better than one large one for patients with more severe heart failure. Referral to a dietitian may be needed.

Patients with heart failure have a terminal illness and may need to be referred to specialist services like palliative care.

The value of nurse-run clinics

Whatever practice nurses undertake in the field of health promotion for patients with chronic diseases, the requirement to produce evidence of its worth remains the same. In fact, the greater the number of opportunities for nurse involvement; the greater the need to use the scarce resources most effectively. This means ensuring that the aims of the clinics are being fulfilled and being able to demonstrate their effectiveness. The practice nurse journals regularly feature inspirational articles by experienced practice nurses, which demonstrate how nurses have improved the health and welfare of their patients.

The way chronic diseases have traditionally been managed is set to change with the advent of *Expert Patients*. The Department of Health has published its vision for the future of chronic disease management[24]. Yet the role of practice nurses in working with patients with chronic conditions has always had this precise intention of helping patients to take control and to self-manage their diseases. This document should be required reading for all practice nurses; it could point the way to developments of the role in the future.

Suggestions for reflection on practice

- Are you able to provide a high-quality chronic disease management service in your practice?
- How do you know whether it is meeting the needs of your patients?

Further reading

Beevers, G., Lip, G. & O'Brien, E. (2000) *ABC of Hypertension* (4th Edn). BMJ Publications, London.

Lindsay, G. & Gaw, A. (eds) (1997) *Coronary Heart Disease Prevention. A handbook for the Health Care Team*. Churchill Livingstone, Edinburgh.

References

1. National Asthma Campaign press release (2001) *National Asthma Campaign. Asthma Audit reveals rise in estimated asthma prevalence – from 3.4 to 5.1 million*. *www.asthma.org.uk/newspr42.html* (accessed 10/10/01).

2. British Thoracic Society (1997) Guidelines on the management of asthma. *Thorax*, **52** (suppl.), S1–21.
3. Kelly, B. (2001) U-turn on steroid dose for asthma guidelines. *Pulse*, **61** (40), 4.
4. British Medical Association and Royal Pharmaceutical Association of Great Britain (2001) *British National Formulary*, 3.1.3 Theopylline. British Medical Association and Royal Pharmaceutical Association, London.
5. Wan, Y. (2000) *Inhaled corticosteroids and growth suppression in children*. Drug Information News. *www.druginfozone.org/news/Mar00/mar_news24/* (accessed 10/10/01).
6. United Nations Environment Programme (1987) *The Montreal Protocol on Substances that Deplete the Ozone Layer*. The Ozone Secretariat. *www.unep.ch/ozone/montreal* (accessed 25/8/01).
7. NICE (2000) *Guidance on use of inhalers for under 5s with Asthma*. National Institute for Clinical Excellence *www.nice.org.uk* (accessed 25/8/01).
8. Office of Population, Censuses and Surveys (1993) *Mortality Statistics, Cause: England and Wales 1992 DH2 (19)*, HMSO, London.
9. British Thoracic Society (1997) BTS guidelines for the management of chronic obstructive airways disease. *Thorax*, **52** (suppl.), S1–32.
10. Bellamy, D. & Booker, R. (2000) *Chronic Obstructive Pulmonary Disease in Primary Care*. Class Publishing, London.
11. Kerstjens, H. & Postma, D. (2000) Chronic obstructive pulmonary disease. *Clinical Evidence*, **3**, 705.
12. World Health Organisation (1999) *Definition, Diagnosis and Classification of Diabetes Mellitus and its Complications: report of a WHO consultation*. World Health Organisation, Department of Noncommunicable Disease Surveillance, Geneva.
13. Diabetes UK (2000) *Understanding Diabetes – Your key to better health*; p. 14. Diabetes UK, London.
14. National Institute for Clinical Excellence (2000) *Guidance on the Use of Rosiglitazone for Type II Diabetes*. National Institute for Clinical Excellence, London.
15. National Institute for Clinical Excellence (2001) *Guidance on the Use of Pioglitazone for Type II Diabetes Mellitus*. National Institute for Clinical Excellence, London.
16. Herman, W. (2000) Glycaemic control in diabetes. *Clinical Evidence*, **3**, 285–9.
17. Diabetes UK (2000) *What Diabetes Care to Expect*. Diabetes UK, London.
18. Diabetes UK (2000) Care recommendation. *Aspirin Treatment in Diabetes*. Diabetes UK, London.
19. British Hypertension Society (1999) Guidelines for the management of hypertension. Report of the 3rd working party of the British Hypertension Society. *Journal of Human Hypertension*, **13**, 569–92.
20. British Hypertension Society (2000) *British Hypertension Society Guidelines for the Management of Hypertension 2000*: Brief summary. *www.hyp.ac.uk/bhs/g12000.htm* (accessed 25/8/01).
21. O'Brien, E., Waeber, B., Parati, G., Taessen, J. & Myers, M. (2001) Blood pressure measuring devices: recommendations of the European Society of Hypertension. *British Medical Journal*, **320**, 1128–34.
22. Department of Health (2000) *National Service Framework for Coronary Heart Disease – Modern Standards and Service Models*. Department of Health, London.
23. Department of Health (2000) *National Service Framework for Cronary Heart Disease – Modern Standards and Service Models*. Department of Health, London.

24. Department of Health (2001) *The Expert Patient: a New Approach to Chronic Disease management for the 21st Century.* Department of Health, London.

Useful addresses and web sites

British Heart Foundation
14 Fitzhardinge Street, London W1H 6DH
Web site: *www.bhf.org.uk*

British Thoracic Society
Web site: *www.brit-thoractic.org.uk*

British Hypertension Society
Web site: *www.hyp.ac.uk*

DTC Primary Care Training Centre
Crow Trees, 27 Town Lane, Idle, Bradford BD10 8 NT
Telephone: 01274 617617
Web site: *www.primarycaretraining.co.uk*

Diabetes UK (Central office)
10 Queen Anne Street, London W1G 9LH
Telephone: 020 7323 1531
Web site: *www.diabetes.org.uk*

General Practitioners in Asthma Group
Web site: *www.gpiag-asthma.org.uk*

National Asthma Campaign
Providence House, Providence Place, London N1 0NT
Telephone: 020 7226 2260
Web site: *www.asthma.org.uk*

National Respiratory Training Centre
The Athenaeum, 10 Church Street, Warwick CV34 4AB
Telephone: 01926 493313
Web site: *www.nartc.org.uk*

Appendices

Appendix 1

Examples of the clinical equipment needed in the nurses' rooms

Examination equipment

  examination couch, paper rolls, pillow, protective pillow covers
  directable, heat filtered lamp
  accurate weighing scales, height measure and body mass index chart
  sphygmomanometer
  stethoscope
  thermometer
  otoscope with aural specula in all sizes
  pen-torch and tongue depressors
  spare batteries and bulbs
  eye chart
  tissues
  examination gloves and jelly
  disposal bags and bins

Clinical test equipment

  urinalysis test strips
  pregnancy tests
  sterile universal containers
  sterile paediatric urine collection bags
  tray with range of pathology blood tubes, alcohol wipes, cotton wool balls, tourniquet,
    needles and vacuum tube holders, small adhesive plasters
  pathology request forms
  blood glucose test strips, lancets and glucose meter with control solution
  sharps bins and yellow bags for clinical waste
  sterile bacterial, endocervical and viral swabs
  vaginal specula, spatulae, endocervical brushes, glass slides, fixative and carrying
    boxes
  adult and paediatric peak flow meters and mouthpieces
  spirometer

charts of normal values
placebo inhaler devices and medication for reversibility tests
carbon monoxide monitor
electrocardiogram machine
Doppler ultrasound
screening audiometer

Equipment for treatment room procedures

Dressings
sterile dressing packs, sterile and unsterile gauze
normal saline sachets/pods
comprehensive range of dressings, bandages and adhesive tapes (see Chapter 5
    under dressings)
skin closure strips and tissue adhesive
plastic bowl for washing feet and legs
emollient creams
dressing scissors
stitch cutters and staple removers
ring cutter
cold-pack for soft-tissue injuries

Ear irrigation
otoscope with spare bulb and batteries
waterproof cape
head light or head mirror and lamp
electric ear syringe
Noots ear tank
Jobson Horne probe
cotton wool
tissues

Nasal examination/treatment
Thudicum nasal specula
Tilley nasal forceps

Minor surgery equipment
trolley
sterile CSSD packs or autoclave and Chaetle forceps
disposable plastic aprons
surgical hand scrub
sterile surgeons' gloves
local anaesthetic injections, plain and with adrenaline
ethyl chloride spray
sterile minor surgery packs or dressing packs

gallipots
povidone iodine skin cleanser
scalpel handles and blades or disposable scalpels
toothed and non-toothed dissecting forceps
straight and curved artery forceps
curette
needle holders
straight and curved scissors
splinter forceps
sinus forceps
nail elevator
specimen containers and formaldehyde solution
cautery
silver nitrate applicators
sterile suture materials
liquid nitrogen or aerosol freezer spray
disposal bags for clinical waste and bag/container for used instruments

If CSSD not used:
washing up liquid and household gloves
ultrasonic bath and enzymatic solution
lubricant spray for instruments

Gynaecological equipment and family planning

vaginal specula – Cusco's small, medium and large and Winterton's (with longer
   blades)
Rampley sponge-holding forceps
Allis tissue forceps
Galabin uterine sound or disposable sounds
Hegar double-ended dilators in range of sizes
8″ artery forceps
Sims uterine scissors
Emmett thread retriever
sterile IUDs and IUSs
sanitary towels and pantie liners

Condoms and diaphragms
   sizing rings for diaphragm
   diaphragms and caps in range of sizes
   range of condoms (if supplied to general practice)
   spermicides for demonstration

Injectables
   medroxyprogesterone acetate
   norethisterone oenanthate (if needed)

Demonstration samples for teaching
   contraceptive pills, condoms, diaphragms, IUDs and implants
   teaching models for IUD, diaphragm and condoms
   instruction leaflets for all methods

Appendix 2

Emergency equipment

Emergency box with syringes, needles and swabs

Drugs, depending on practice policy:
   atropine sulphate 600 mg
   benzylpenicillin 600 mg and water for injection
   chlorpheniramine 10 mg
   diclofenac 75 mg
   epinephrine (adrenaline) 1:1000
   frusemide 20 mg
   glucagon 1 mg in 1 ml
   glucose 50% solution 50 ml for IV use, follow by normal saline solution
   hydrocortisone 100 mg
   naloxone 400 mcg
   procyclidine 10 mg
   terbutaline 500 mcg

Other drugs:
   aspirin 300 mg chewable tablets
   glyceryl trinitrate spray
   prednisolone 5 mg tablets/dispersible tablets
   rectal diazepam 5 mg

adult and child resuscitation masks with one-way valves or Ambu bag
oxygen cylinder and giving set
suction
intravenous needles, giving set, and infusion solution
adult and paediatric laryngoscopes and range of endotracheal tubes (if clinicians in
   practice able to use safely)
defibrillator (not commonly kept in urban practices, but essential in rural practices)

Emergency asthma treatment

large volume spacer and salbutamol inhaler
nebuliser with supply of single-patient-use nebulising kits with mouthpieces and
   adult and child masks
salbutamol 2.5 mg and 5 mg nebules
budesonide 0.5 in 2 ml nebules
impratropium bromide nebules

Eye treatment

magnifying head lens (Loup)
normal saline for irrigation
eye drops:
– Fluorescein 1%
– Amethocaine 1%
– Chloromycetin (chloramphenicol)
blue/green light torch or opthalmoscope to examine fluorescein-stained eyes
tipped applicators

Appendix 3

Guidelines for patients with diabetes on coping with sickness

If you are unwell, or have a gastric upset, your diabetes is likely to be affected. The following guidelines should be followed:

- Do not stop your insulin or tablets even if you do not feel like eating. Consult your doctor or diabetes nurse in case your dosage needs to be adjusted.
- Check your diabetes control at least four times a day – blood or urine test.
- Test your urine for ketones if you are treated with insulin.
- Drink plenty of fluids.
- If unable to eat your normal meals take regular measured amounts of drinks containing concentrated carbohydrates, e.g.
  - 50 ml Lucozade
  - 100 ml natural unsweetened fruit juice
  - 200 ml milk.
- Consult your doctor or diabetes nurse if:
  - unable to keep fluids down
  - there are large amounts of ketones in your urine
  - your blood sugar control remains unstable.

Index